Reproduction in Transgender and Nonbinary Individuals

Molly B. Moravek • Gene de Haan
Editors

Reproduction in Transgender and Nonbinary Individuals

A Clinical Guide

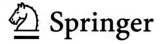

Editors
Molly B. Moravek
Department of Obstetrics & Gynecology
University of Michigan–Ann Arbor
Ann Arbor, MI, USA

Gene de Haan
Obstetrics and Gynecology
Northwest Permanente
Portland, OR, USA

ISBN 978-3-031-14935-1   ISBN 978-3-031-14933-7   (eBook)
https://doi.org/10.1007/978-3-031-14933-7

© The Editor(s) (if applicable) and The Author(s), under exclusive license to Springer Nature Switzerland AG 2023

This work is subject to copyright. All rights are solely and exclusively licensed by the Publisher, whether the whole or part of the material is concerned, specifically the rights of translation, reprinting, reuse of illustrations, recitation, broadcasting, reproduction on microfilms or in any other physical way, and transmission or information storage and retrieval, electronic adaptation, computer software, or by similar or dissimilar methodology now known or hereafter developed.

The use of general descriptive names, registered names, trademarks, service marks, etc. in this publication does not imply, even in the absence of a specific statement, that such names are exempt from the relevant protective laws and regulations and therefore free for general use.

The publisher, the authors, and the editors are safe to assume that the advice and information in this book are believed to be true and accurate at the date of publication. Neither the publisher nor the authors or the editors give a warranty, expressed or implied, with respect to the material contained herein or for any errors or omissions that may have been made. The publisher remains neutral with regard to jurisdictional claims in published maps and institutional affiliations.

This Springer imprint is published by the registered company Springer Nature Switzerland AG
The registered company address is: Gewerbestrasse 11, 6330 Cham, Switzerland

Contents

**1 Introduction to the Demographics and Reproductive Health
Needs of Transgender and Nonbinary People** 1
Halley P. Crissman and Gene de Haan

2 Overview of Gender-Affirming Therapy 9
Chelsea N. Fortin and John F. Randolph

3 Effects of Masculinizing Therapy on Reproductive Capacity 33
Hadrian M. Kinnear and Molly B. Moravek

**4 Fertility and Fertility Preservation in Transmasculine
Individuals** 49
Brett Stark, Viji Sundaram, and Evelyn Mok-Lin

5 Fertility and Fertility Preservation for Transfeminine Adults 59
Jessica Long, James F. Smith, and Amanda J. Adeleye

**6 Obstetric, Antenatal, and Postpartum Care for
Transgender and Nonbinary People** 75
Gnendy Indig, Sebastian Ramos, and Daphna Stroumsa

7 Fertility Preservation in Transgender and Non-binary Youth 97
Rebecca M. Harris, Michelle Bayefsky, Gwendolyn P. Quinn,
and Leena Nahata

**8 Non-procreative Reproductive Issues and Sexual Function
in Transmasculine Individuals** 109
Frances Grimstad

**9 Non-procreative Reproductive Issues and Sexual Function
in Transfeminine Individuals** 129
Kyle R. Latack, Shane D. Morrison, and Miriam Hadj-Moussa

10 Psychosocial Aspects of Reproduction in Transgender and Non-binary Individuals 141
Mariam Maksutova and Angela K. Lawson

11 Legal Considerations 153
Will Halm, Eliseo Arebalos, Catherine B. McGowan,
Rachael J. Bailey, and Malina Simard-Halm

12 Ethical Considerations for Transgender and Non-Binary Reproduction 163
Lisa Campo-Engelstein and Rebecca M. Permar

13 Creating Inclusive, Gender Affirming Clinical Environments 177
Jen Hastings, Ben Geilhufe, J. M. Jaffe, Jenna Rapues,
and Colt St. Amand

Index 209

Chapter 1
Introduction to the Demographics and Reproductive Health Needs of Transgender and Nonbinary People

Halley P. Crissman and Gene de Haan

Contemporary estimates suggest that approximately 0.5–0.6% of US adults identify as transgender [1, 2]. This is likely a gross underestimate, as we will explore in more detail later in this chapter. Transgender is a term individuals may use to describe their gender identity when their gender does not align with that typically expected by their culture based on their sex assigned at birth, whereas the term cisgender is used to describe people whose gender identity aligns with cultural expectations for their sex assigned at birth. Often cultural expectations are cisnormative and assume a gender binary—that people assigned female sex at birth will identify and express themselves as girls and women, and that people assigned male sex at birth will identify and express themselves as boys and men. However, gender is a dynamic socially constructed spectrum, and many people's gender identities do not fit neatly into the dichotomies of feminine and masculine, or women and men. Individuals with a gender identity outside of the binary may or may not identify under the umbrella of transgender and may describe their identities with terms including nonbinary, genderqueer, or gender expansive. For the purposes of this text, we will use the phrase transgender and nonbinary (TGNB) as an overarching term to describe non-cisgender people.

Understanding the demographics and health outcomes of gender diverse populations is complicated by the frequent conflation of sex and gender. Sex refers to one's reproductive organs, native hormones, and chromosomes, and is typically assigned at birth based on the appearance of the genitals. Gender identity refers to one's internal sense of being a man or boy, a woman or girl, or another gender. Gaps in

---

H. P. Crissman (✉)
Department of Obstetrics and Gynecology, University of Michigan, Ann Arbor, MI, USA
e-mail: hcrissma@med.umich.edu

G. de Haan
Department of Obstetrics and Gynecology, NW Permanente, Portland, OR, USA
e-mail: gene.dehaan@kp.org

© The Author(s), under exclusive license to Springer Nature Switzerland AG 2023
M. B. Moravek, G. de Haan (eds.), *Reproduction in Transgender and Nonbinary Individuals*, https://doi.org/10.1007/978-3-031-14933-7_1

national probability data on reproductive health among gender minority populations are in large part due to widespread conflation of sex and gender. Use of single-item questions regarding sex or gender in surveys, rather than the recommended two-step approach to determining sex assigned at birth and gender identity, result in an assumption of cisgender identities and an inability to identify gender diverse people [3]. Many surveys ask participants for their "gender" and give options such as male or female. Single-item questions such as this leave it unclear whether the survey is truly interested in one's gender or one's sex—and fail to acknowledge and capture the existence of TGNB people. For example, the National Survey of Family Growth (NSFG), a large annual survey by the Centers for Disease Control and Prevention (CDC) regarding family life, and reproductive health including pregnancy, infertility, and use of contraception, fails to differentiate between sex and gender. The NSFG provides participants with either a male or female questionnaire based on the "gender" of members of a household (as identified by the head of household), resulting in conflation of sex and gender, and a missed opportunity to gather information about the reproductive health of TGNB people.

In 2011, the Institute of Medicine summarized the data on transgender people in the USA as "sorely lacking." [4] Most research regarding TGNB people to date has utilized convenience and clinical samples, rather than population representative samples. Currently, the best estimates regarding the prevalence of TGNB identities in the United States come from the CDC Behavioral Risk Factor Surveillance Symptom which for the first time in 2014 gave states the option to include questions regarding gender identity; survey respondents in 19 states and territories were asked "do you consider yourself to be transgender?" allowing researchers to calculate a multi-state estimate of the prevalence of transgender identity using probability data for the first time [1, 2]. Based on this data it estimated that approximately 0.5–0.6% of adults, or 1.0–1.4 million people, identify as transgender in the United States [1, 2]. Notably, these methods exclude non-cisgender people who do not identify as transgender, and individuals who did not disclose their identity to the interviewer. More recent data suggests transgender identity is more common among youth in the United States. In 2017, 10 states and multiple urban areas collected data on transgender identity as part of the Youth Risk Behavior Survey [5]. Overall, 1.8% of youth in grades 9–12 self-identified as being transgender, suggesting a larger population of openly TGNB identified people in the next generation—and a sizeable population of young people in need of comprehensive healthcare [5]. Forthcoming data from the first US national probability sample of transgender individuals via TransPop Study should aid significantly in advancing our understanding of the demographic parameters and basic health outcomes of TGNB people in the USA, but is not a substitution for the need for two-step sex and gender questions in surveys broadly.

Available data suggest some demographic differences when comparing the TGNB population to the general adult US population. Adults who identify as transgender are more racially and ethnically diverse than the general adult US population; multi-state data suggests 55% of transgender adults in the USA identify as White, 16% as African-American or Black, 21% as Latinx or Hispanic, and 8% as

1 Introduction to the Demographics and Reproductive Health Needs of Transgender... 3

another race or ethnicity (compared to rates of 66%, 12%, 15%, and 8% respectively in the general adult US population) [2, 6]. By one multi-state estimate of transgender-identified adults, the prevalence of transfeminine identities (0.28%) were more common than transmasculine identities (0.16%) or identifying as gender nonconforming (0.08%) [2]. The adult transgender-identified population appears similar to the US general population in terms of age, urban or rural living situation, and marital status [2, 7, 8]. However, consistent with the expected sequela of discrimination and marginalization, from a socioeconomic standpoint, transgender-identified adults are more likely to be below the poverty line, and are less likely to have attended college [2]. Additionally, transgender adults in the USA are less likely to have health insurance coverage (18.0 vs 11.0%) [8].

Beyond disparities in health insurance coverage, TGNB people face significant barriers to health and healthcare including stigma, and institutional and interpersonal gender discrimination (affecting housing, employment, criminal justice system engagement, insurance, and social support access) [9–14]. Accessing reproductive and sexual health may raise unique challenges and barriers for TGNB people. In particular, the gendered environment and intimate nature of sexual and reproductive healthcare—conceptualized and often labeled "women's health"—may make TGNB people hesitant or dysphoric in seeking care [15, 16]. Moreover, providers may lack cultural and medical competency in caring for the reproductive and sexual healthcare needs of TGNB people, and patients may face trans-specific insurance barriers to care (such as the requirement for letters of mental health support for coverage of some services, or insurance processing challenges for sex-specific services) [16, 17].

Much of the reproductive health research regarding TGNB people historically focused on high-risk sexual activity and the risk of HIV. This is not without reason—the data on HIV among transgender adults in the USA are staggering—an estimated 1.4% of transgender US adults have HIV, compared with 0.3% of the general population [13]. Moreover, there are significant racial disparities in these rates—by self-reporting an estimated 1 in 5 Black transwomen are living with HIV [13]. However, for TGNB people, like all people, there is far more to sex and intimacy than risk of infection. TGNB people have diverse sexualities, sexual health practices, and reproductive health needs.

For some gender diverse people, being involved in reproduction is core to their sense of self, and desires for family building. Often people invoke a simplistic understanding of transgender identity—a narrative that TGNB individuals are "trapped in the wrong body." Many thus erroneously assume that all TGNB individuals, particularly those that transition with medical assistance, reject their reproductive organs and the reproductive capacity of their natal sex organs. Sterility of TGNB has in fact been not only assumed, but it has been legislated by numerous countries as a requirement for legal recognition of the gender identity of TGNB people—a practice which was ruled to be a human rights violation by the European Court of Human Rights in 2017 (https://tgeu.org/echr_end-sterilisation/).

Just like not all TGNB individuals undergo hormone or surgical interventions, not all gender diverse people feel at odds with their natal reproductive capacity [18].

In a study of TGNB youth, nearly half were interested in having children, and 36% were interested in biologic fertility [19]. Biologic fertility may be in the form of contributing gametes and/or carrying a pregnancy [20, 21]. Among TGNB people who carry pregnancies or engage in assisted reproduction, some describe reproduction as congruent with their gender identity, while others describe it as gender incongruent but necessary in achieving parenthood [18, 22]. Those requiring assisted reproduction describe going to great lengths, and in many cases incredible resilience, in overcoming challenges including transphobia from staff, and dysphoria with exams, hormones, and bleeding, all to achieve the goal of a biologic child [23].

Many TGNB people do not receive counseling, or acknowledgement of family planning and their reproductive capacity, by their healthcare providers. Most patients report they were not asked about fertility or family planning prior to initiating gender-affirming medical therapies, despite the potential implications of these therapies on fertility [19, 24]. Studies suggest that large minorities of TGNB people assigned female or male sex at birth, who were not offered fertility preservation prior to sterilization surgeries, would have considered it if it had been presented as an option [25, 26]. Beyond the implications for sterilizing procedures, failure to recognize TGNB people as engaging in sex with pregnancy potential and reproduction has downstream implications for many aspects of gender-affirming care. For example, transmasculine individuals in one study universally noted feeling unable to ask their top (mastectomy) surgeon about the potential implications of future pregnancy on their top surgery outcome and lactation—they described feeling that they had to stick to a narrative of "trapped in the wrong body" to avoid jeopardizing their ability to get surgery [27]. Moreover, the assumption of reproduction as restricted to cisgender people contributes to internalized transphobia, discrimination, and violence against TGNB people engaged in reproduction, and has negative implications for access to comprehensive sexual and reproductive healthcare (including contraception, comprehensive sexual health screenings, pre-conception care, fertility services, pregnancy care, abortion, postpartum services as well as other gender-affirming surgical care).

For TGNB who do not desire conception or wish to delay conception and engage in sex with pregnancy potential, access to contraception is essential [28]. While rates of engagement in sex with pregnancy potential are not well documented in TGNB populations, TGNB people have diverse sexualities [8]. One recent study of transmasculine people found that more than 50% reported having a partner who was assigned male sex at birth in the last 12 months [21]. A minority of TGNB people have had a sterilizing surgery; in a large national survey of transgender adults 11% of transgender women had undergone an orchiectomy and 14% of transgender men had undergone a hysterectomy—comparable to the 18.9% of females in the general population ages 15–44 years old who report having had either a hysterectomy or other sterilization procedure [13, 29]. Findings from administrative claims data suggests transmasculine people are less likely to be prescribed oral contraceptive pills, or long-acting reversible contraception, than cisgender women [30]. Gender-affirming hormones are not recommended or approved as contraception, despite misconceptions they may be used as such [21, 24, 31]. In one study, 16% of transmasculine individuals reported using testosterone as contraception, and 5.5% of respondents reported that their healthcare provider told them that testosterone was a contraceptive, suggesting gaps in both patient and provider knowledge [24]. While there is currently a lack of data regarding conception rates while using testosterone, pregnancies in the setting of testosterone-induced amenorrhea have been reported [20, 24]. Potential underutilization of contraception with concomitant testosterone use is problematic given concerns for unmet need for contraception, risk of exacerbation of gender dysphoria in the setting of pregnancy, barriers to accessing pregnancy care, and the known masculinizing effects of testosterone on XX fetuses [18, 32, 33]. Particularly in the setting of drastric disparities geographically in access to abortion care in the wake of the Supreme Court's *Dobbs* decision, it is critical that gender diverse people get accurate information about family building, fertility, and contraception, and that remaining abortion care is inclusive and accessible for people of all gender. In the setting of pregnancy, existing binary gender classification systems and practitioners' cisnormative assumptions may cause them to fail to recognize pregnancy in a TGNB patient, particularly those which are unplanned, placing the pregnant person and fetus at increased risk of unrecognized pregnancy-related morbidities [34].

While barriers make accessing reproductive and sexual healthcare more difficult for TGNB people, people of all genders need and deserve sexual and reproductive healthcare. We as providers have a duty to ensure patients receive high quality care regardless of gender. Though the status quo of reproductive and sexual healthcare provision is not adequately meeting the needs of gender diverse people, positive change is possible through advocacy, education, and policy change. Advocates and researchers are increasingly calling out the unacceptable disparities and barriers to reproductive healthcare for TGNB people, and are advocating for the disentangling of sex and gender in research and clinical care [15, 35–37]. While medical education is currently insufficient, provider training is associated with reduced provider transphobia [38, 39]. Moreover, though complicated by political turnover, rules like Section 1557 of the Affordable Care Act have pushed insurance companies to move away from blanket exclusions in gender-affirming care (https://www.hhs.gov/sites/default/files/section-1557-final-rule-faqs.pdf) [36]. With education, commitment to gender non-discrimination policies and practices, the sexual and reproductive healthcare for all people can be enhanced through gender-affirming care.

References

1. Flores AR, Herman JL, Gates GJ, Brown TNT. How many adults identify as transgender in the United States? *The Williams Institute*; 2016. p. 13.
2. Crissman HP, Berger MB, Graham LF, Dalton VK. Transgender demographics: a household probability sample of US adults, 2014. Am J Public Health. 2017;107(2):213–5.

3. Gender Identity in Surveillance Group. Best practices for asking questions to identify transgender and other gender minority respondents on population-based surveys. Published online 2014. http://williamsinstitute.law.ucla.edu/wp-content/uploads/geniuss-report-sep-2014.pdf
4. Institute of Medicine (U.S.). *The health of lesbian, gay, bisexual, and transgender people: building a foundation for better understanding.* National Academies Press; 2011.
5. Johns MM, Lowry R, Andrzejewski J, et al. Transgender identity and experiences of violence victimization, substance use, suicide risk, and sexual risk behaviors among high school students — 19 States and large Urban School Districts, 2017. MMWR Morbidity and Mortality Weekly Report. 2019;68(3):67–71. https://doi.org/10.15585/mmwr.mm6803a3.
6. Flores AR, Brown TNT, Herman JL. Race and ethnicity of adults who identify as transgender in the United States. Los Angeles, CA: Williams Institute, UCLA School of Law; 2016. p. 15.
7. Herman JL, Flores AR, Brown TN, Wilson BD, Conron KJ. Age of individuals who identify as transgender in the United States. The Williams Institute. 2017. Accessed October 13, 2017. https://williamsinstitute.law.ucla.edu/wp-content/uploads/TransAgeReport.pdf
8. Meyer IH, Brown TN, Herman JL, Reisner SL, Bockting WO. Demographic characteristics and health status of transgender adults in select US regions: behavioral risk factor surveillance system, 2014. Am J Public Health. 2017;107(4):582–9.
9. Bauer GR, Zong X, Scheim AI, Hammond R, Thind A. Factors Impacting Transgender Patients' Discomfort with Their Family Physicians: A Respondent-Driven Sampling Survey. Clark JL, ed. PLOS ONE. 2015;10(12):e0145046. https://doi.org/10.1371/journal.pone.0145046.
10. Bockting WO, Robinson BE, Rosser BRS. Transgender HIV prevention: a qualitative needs assessment. AIDS Care. 1998;10(4):505–25. https://doi.org/10.1080/09540129850124028.
11. Cruz TM. Assessing access to care for transgender and gender nonconforming people: a consideration of diversity in combating discrimination. Soc Sci Med. 2014;110:65–73. https://doi.org/10.1016/j.socscimed.2014.03.032.
12. Grant JM, Mottet LA, Tanis JJ, Min D. Injustice at every turn: a report of the national transgender discrimination survey. 2011. Accessed September 25, 2017. http://www.academia.edu/download/31122982/NTDS_Report.pdf
13. James SE, Herman JL, Rankin S, Keisling M, Mottet L, Anafi M. The Report of the 2015 U.S. Transgender Survey; 2016.
14. Seelman KL, Colón-Diaz MJP, LeCroix RH, Xavier-Brier M, Kattari L. Transgender non-inclusive healthcare and delaying care because of fear: connections to general health and mental health among transgender adults. Transgender Health. 2017;2(1):17–28. https://doi.org/10.1089/trgh.2016.0024.
15. Stroumsa D, Wu JP. Welcoming transgender and nonbinary patients: expanding the language of "women's health". Am J Obstetr Gynecol. 2018;219(6):585.e1–5. https://doi.org/10.1016/j.ajog.2018.09.018.
16. Moseson H, Zazanis N, Goldberg E, et al. The imperative for transgender and gender nonbinary inclusion: beyond Women's health. Obstet Gynecol. 2020;135(5):1059–68. https://doi.org/10.1097/AOG.0000000000003816.
17. Unger CA. Care of the Transgender Patient: a survey of gynecologists' current knowledge and practice. J Women's Health. 2015;24(2):114–8. https://doi.org/10.1089/jwh.2014.4918.
18. Ellis SA, Wojnar DM, Pettinato M. Conception, pregnancy, and birth experiences of male and gender variant gestational parents: It's how we could have a family. J Midwifery Womens Health. 2015;60(1):62–9. https://doi.org/10.1111/jmwh.12213.
19. Chen D, Matson M, Macapagal K, et al. Attitudes toward fertility and reproductive health among transgender and gender-nonconforming adolescents. J Adolesc Health. 2018;63(1):62–8. https://doi.org/10.1016/j.jadohealth.2017.11.306.
20. Light AD, Obedin-Maliver J, Sevelius JM, Kerns JL. Transgender men who experienced pregnancy after female-to-male gender transitioning. Obstetr Gynecol. 2014;124(6):1120–7. https://doi.org/10.1097/AOG.0000000000000540.
21. Stark B, Hughto JMW, Charlton BM, Deutsch MB, Potter J, Reisner SL. The contraceptive and reproductive history and planning goals of trans masculine adults: a mixed methods study. Contraception. 2019; https://doi.org/10.1016/j.contraception.2019.07.146.

1 Introduction to the Demographics and Reproductive Health Needs of Transgender...

22. Hoffkling A, Obedin-Maliver J, Sevelius J. From erasure to opportunity: a qualitative study of the experiences of transgender men around pregnancy and recommendations for providers. BMC Pregnancy Childbirth. 2017;17(S2) https://doi.org/10.1186/s12884-017-1491-5.

23. Armuand G, Dhejne C, Olofsson JI, Rodriguez-Wallberg KA. Transgender men's experiences of fertility preservation: a qualitative study. Hum Reprod. 2017;32(2):383–90. https://doi.org/10.1093/humrep/dew323.

24. Light A, Wang L-F, Zeymo A, Gomez-Lobo V. Family planning and contraception use in transgender men. Contraception. 2018;98(4):266–9. https://doi.org/10.1016/j.contraception.2018.06.006.

25. Wierckx K, Van Caenegem E, Elaut E, et al. Quality of life and sexual health after sex reassignment surgery in transsexual men. J Sex Med. 2011;8(12):3379–88. https://doi.org/10.1111/j.1743-6109.2011.02348.x.

26. De Sutter P, Verschoor A, Hotimsky A, Kira K. The desire to have children and the preservation of fertility in transsexual women: A survey. Int J Transgend. 2002;6(3) No Pagination Specified-No Pagination Specified.

27. MacDonald T, Noel-Weiss J, West D, et al. Transmasculine individuals' experiences with lactation, chestfeeding, and gender identity: a qualitative study. BMC Pregnancy Childbirth. 2016;16:1. https://doi.org/10.1186/s12884-016-0907-y.

28. Bonnington A, Dianat S, Kerns J, et al. Society of Family Planning clinical recommendations: contraceptive counseling for transgender and gender diverse people who were female sex assigned at birth. Contraception. 2020;102(2):70–82. https://doi.org/10.1016/j.contraception.2020.04.001.

29. Percent Distribution of Women Aged 15–49, by Current Contraceptive Status: United States, 2015–2017. National Survey of Family Growth, 2015–2017 Accessed January 9, 2020. https://www.cdc.gov/nchs/data/databriefs/db327_tables-508.pdf#page=2

30. Crissman et al. Leveraging administrative claims to understand dispartities in gender minority health: contraceptive use patterns among transgender and nonbinary people. LGBT Health. 2022.

31. Schwartz AR, Russell K, Gray BA. Approaches to vaginal bleeding and contraceptive counseling in transgender and gender nonbinary patients. Obstetr Gynecol. 2019;1 https://doi.org/10.1097/AOG.0000000000003308.

32. Wingo E, Ingraham N, Roberts SCM. Reproductive health care priorities and barriers to effective care for LGBTQ people assigned female at birth: a qualitative study. Womens Health Issues. 2018;28(4):350–7. https://doi.org/10.1016/j.whi.2018.03.002.

33. Wolf CJ. Effects of prenatal testosterone propionate on the sexual development of male and female rats: a dose-response study. Toxicol Sci. 2002;65(1):71–86. https://doi.org/10.1093/toxsci/65.1.71.

34. Stroumsa D, Roberts EFS, Kinnear H, Harris LH. The power and limits of classification — a 32-year-old man with abdominal pain. N Engl J Med. 2019;380(20):1885–8. https://doi.org/10.1056/NEJMp1811491.

35. Shteyler VM, Clarke JA, Adashi EY. Failed assignments — rethinking sex designations on birth certificates. N Engl J Med. 2020;383(25):2399–401. https://doi.org/10.1056/NEJMp2025974.

36. Stroumsa D, Kirkland AR. Health coverage and care for transgender people — threats and opportunities. N Engl J Med. 2020;383(25):2397–9.

37. American College of Obstetricians and Gynecologists. Committee opinion: health care for transgender individuals. Number 512. Published online December 2011.

38. Braun HM, Garcia-Grossman IR, Quiñones-Rivera A, Deutsch MB. Outcome and impact evaluation of a transgender health course for health profession students. LGBT Health. 2017;4(1):55–61. https://doi.org/10.1089/lgbt.2016.0119.

39. Stroumsa D, Shires DA, Richardson CR, Jaffee KD, Woodford MR. Transphobia rather than education predicts provider knowledge of transgender health care. Med Educ. 2019;21 https://doi.org/10.1111/medu.13796.

Chapter 2
Overview of Gender-Affirming Therapy

Chelsea N. Fortin and John F. Randolph

Introduction

Transgender and nonbinary (TGNB) individuals often seek gender-affirming therapy to harmonize their external appearance and affirmed gender, thereby alleviating feelings of gender dysphoria. These therapies can include hormonal therapies and surgical interventions. According to the National Transgender Discrimination Survey Report, 80% of transgender individuals have utilized, or would like to utilize, gender-affirming hormones [1]. Furthermore, an estimated 25–35% of transgender individuals have undergone gender-affirming surgery [2, 3]. As the number of TGNB individuals seeking these therapies continues to grow [4], it is increasingly important for healthcare providers to be informed of the basic tenets of gender-affirming care.

Initiation of Hormone Therapy

Initiation of gender-affirming hormone therapy is often the first step towards reconciling the incongruence between a transgender individual's external appearance and identified gender identity. Individualizing the approach to hormone therapy is essential, so that the patient's goals are achieved safely and effectively. This should be a shared decision-making process between patients and providers. Prior to hormone initiation, a thorough history should be obtained to explore pertinent medical, psychological, and social issues [5, 6]. Patients should be counseled on the expected

---

C. N. Fortin (✉) · J. F. Randolph
Department of Obstetrics and Gynecology, Division of Reproductive Endocrinology and Infertility, University of Michigan, Ann Arbor, MI, USA
e-mail: chfo@med.umich.edu; jfrandol@med.umich.edu

© The Author(s), under exclusive license to Springer Nature Switzerland AG 2023
M. B. Moravek, G. de Haan (eds.), *Reproduction in Transgender and Nonbinary Individuals*, https://doi.org/10.1007/978-3-031-14933-7_2

timeline for physical changes as well as potential risks of hormone therapy [6]. This should include a discussion on the impact of treatments on fertility and options for fertility preservation. Baseline laboratory studies should be checked, including hemoglobin/hematocrit prior to masculinizing hormone therapy and a metabolic panel prior to feminizing hormone therapy [5–7]. Individuals should have full capacity to make informed medical decisions, and informed consent should be obtained prior to initiating hormone therapy.

Masculinizing Therapies

Hormone Therapies

Masculinizing hormone therapy induces the development of male secondary sex characteristics and suppresses female secondary sex characteristics, typically with the use of testosterone [8]. Several different testosterone formulations exist, with no evidence to suggest superiority of one formulation over another [6]. A comparison of transgender men using short-acting intramuscular, long-acting intramuscular, or transdermal testosterone found equivalent satisfaction rates at 1 year of use [9]. Selection should take into account cost, safety, availability, and patient preference.

Medications and Regimens (Table 2.1)

Testosterone cypionate and testosterone enanthate are the most commonly used testosterone formulations in the United States [10]. These agents, classified as testosterone esters, are administered at weekly or biweekly intervals [8]. Weekly dosing is often preferred, as testosterone levels show less fluctuation, resulting in improved stability in sexual function and mood [23]. Compared with patients using other testosterone formulations, patients using parenteral therapy tend to achieve higher testosterone levels more quickly [6]. Testosterone esters can also be administered subcutaneously with similar outcomes to intramuscular injections. Although this route of administration is not currently approved by the US Food and Drug Administration (FDA), studies have found it to be well-tolerated and as effective as intramuscular administration [11, 12]. Although the time to peak testosterone concentration may be longer with subcutaneous compared with intramuscular administration, the peak concentration reached appears to be equivalent [24].

Testosterone undecanoate is a longer-acting parenteral agent that maintains stable serum testosterone concentrations over a 12 week period [13]. Due to rare reports of anaphylaxis and pulmonary oil microemboli, the FDA requires that prescribers enroll in the Risk Evaluation and Mitigation Strategy program [6]. Testosterone undecanoate recently became available in the United States as an oral preparation [25]. While an oral formulation is a seemingly attractive option, in reality it is rarely used, as it is dosed thrice daily and is ineffective at suppressing

2 Overview of Gender-Affirming Therapy

Table 2.1 Overview of gender-affirming hormone therapy regimens [5, 6, 10–22]

Medication	Route	Typical dose	Pros/Cons	Notes
Feminizing[a]				
Estrogens				
17-β estradiol	PO	Initial: 2 mg daily Maintenance: 6–8 mg daily	• Low cost • No injection needed • Higher risk of VTE	• Use divided dosing if total dose >2 mg • Can also give SL (decrease dose)
Conjugated estrogens	PO	Initial: 1.25–2.5 mg daily Maintenance: 5–7.5 mg daily	• No injection needed • Higher risk of VTE • Cannot monitor E2 levels	
Estradiol patch[b]	TD	Initial: 0.025–0.05 mg daily Maintenance: 0.1–0.2 mg daily	• Lower risk of VTE • Uniform E2 levels • No injection needed • Costly • Skin irritation	• Use if increased risk of VTE • Patch changed every 3–5 days
Estradiol valerate	IM	Initial: 5–10 mg weekly Maintenance: 10–20 mg weekly	• Low cost • Injection • Peaks/troughs in E2 levels	• To dose every other week, double dosage
Anti-androgens				
Spironolactone	PO	Initial: 50 mg daily Maintenance: 100 mg BID	• Low cost • Risk of hyperkalemia	• Must monitor blood pressure and potassium levels
Finasteride	PO	1–5 mg daily	• Benefits for hair and skin	
Bicalutamide	PO	50 mg daily	• Risk of hepatotoxicity	
Cyproterone acetate	PO	Initial: 25 mg daily Maintenance: 50 mg daily	• Risk of hepatotoxicity	• Not available in USA
Progestins				
Medroxyprogesterone acetate	IM	150 mg every 3 months	• Limited evidence • May increase risk of VTE, breast cancer, depression, weight gain	• Not recommended by Endocrine Society
Micronized progesterone	PO	100–200 mg QHS	• Limited evidence • May increase risk of VTE, breast cancer, depression, weight gain	• Not recommended by Endocrine Society

(continued)

Table 2.1 (continued)

Medication	Route	Typical dose	Pros/Cons	Notes
Masculinizing[a]				
Testosterone cypionate/ enanthate	IM	50–100 mg weekly	• Low cost • Infrequent dosing • Peaks/troughs in T levels	• To dose every other week, double dosage • Can also give SQ (not FDA approved)
Testosterone undecanoate	IM	1000 mg every 12 weeks	• Longer-acting • Risk of POME • Costly	• Requires REMS to prescribe
	PO	40–80 mg TID	• No injection needed • Frequent dosing • Inconsistent T levels	
Testosterone gel (1%)[b]	TD	50–100 mg daily	• No injection needed • Uniform T levels • Costly • Skin irritation • Transfer to others • Daily application	• Pump or packet form
Testosterone patch[b]	TD	2–8 mg daily	• No injection needed • Uniform T levels • Costly • Skin irritation • Daily application	• 2 mg or 4 mg patches

Adapted from: Fortin, C.N., Moravek, M.B. Medical Transition for Gender Diverse Patients. *Curr Obstet Gynecol Rep* 9, 166–177 (2020)

E2 estradiol, *GnRH* gonadotropin releasing hormone, *IM* intramuscular, *PO* oral, *POME* pulmonary oil microembolism, *QHS* every night at bedtime, *REMS* risk evaluation and mitigation strategy, *SL* sublingual, *SQ* subcutaneous, *T* testosterone, *TID* three times daily, *TD* transdermal, *US* United States, *VTE* venous thromboembolism

[a]The recommended dosing regimen can be modified for nonbinary patients if milder masculinization is desired

[b]Consider higher doses if more adipose tissue

menses due to variable serum testosterone levels [10, 14]. For patients who are unable or unwilling to self-administer injections, transdermal formulations can be considered. These formulations, which include testosterone gels and patches, are often costly, and can potentially cause skin irritation or transfer of the gel onto close contacts [10]. Serum testosterone concentrations tend to be lower in patients using transdermal formulations, which can slow the virilization process and ineffectively suppress menses [26].

Adjunctive medications may be considered in those patients who do not achieve menstrual suppression with testosterone alone [5, 8, 10]. These medications are also useful for patients who request menstrual suppression prior to initiating treatment with testosterone or who are not planning to initiate testosterone therapy [27]. The two most commonly used agents are progestins and gonadotropin releasing hormone (GnRH) agonists [5, 10]. GnRH agonists, such as leuprolide acetate, are effective but often cost-prohibitive, cannot be used long-term, and have significant side effects [6].

Expected Physical Changes

Patients should be counseled that the majority of physical changes should be expected within 2 years of initiating treatment, although the exact timeframe can vary [5, 8, 26]. The extent of physical change is also variable [5]. There is insufficient evidence to reliably predict an individual's response to treatment based on patient-specific characteristics such as age or body mass index (BMI) [5]. Typically, one of the first changes seen is deepening of the voice, which occurs at six to 12 weeks [15]. Prior to initiating testosterone therapy, it is important for patients to understand that testosterone-induced vocal cord changes are irreversible, even with discontinuation of treatment [15, 16]. Studies of long-term testosterone users have demonstrated their voices to be indistinguishable from those of cisgender men [16, 28]. Another physical change considered irreversible is clitoral enlargement [8], which occurs one to 6 months after initiating treatment [5] and can cause clitoral pain [29]. The maximum clitoral length achieved can vary [5], averaging 4.6 cm 1–2 years of treatment [15, 30]. Many transmasculine people consider menstrual suppression the most desired effect of hormone therapy [10]. Cessation of menses will occur within 6 months of treatment for the majority of patients [8, 30]. If menstruation is still occurring at 6 months, further evaluation is warranted (See Chap. 8).

Several other changes will take place after the first 6 months of treatment. The development of acne typically peaks around 6 months of treatment and tends to lessen with time [8, 10, 31]. Although acne is a very common effect of testosterone therapy, very few transmasculine individuals develop moderate or severe acne [29]. Changes in body composition also start within 6 months of hormone therapy initiation and include an increase in muscle mass and visceral fat and decrease in subcutaneous fat [8, 30, 32, 33]. Some studies have found that transmasculine people gain weight while on testosterone therapy, thought to be a result of increased fat-free mass at the expense of fat mass [34–37]. Alternatively, other studies have reported no change in BMI [38, 39]. The extent to which these changes occur will depend largely on the individual's activity level [5]. Height will not be affected if treatment is initiated after puberty [6]. Atrophy of breast tissue may also occur during this period [5].

Patients also typically experience changes in hair growth and distribution within the first 6 months of treatment. This process, however, can take several years to complete [5]. The progression of terminal hair growth typically follows the same pattern seen in cisgender pubertal boys: (1) upper lip, (2) cheeks, (3) pubic area, (4) chin and neck, (5) limbs and chest [15]. The growth of facial and body hair occurs more quickly than does the loss of scalp hair [5]. The processes of terminal hair growth and scalp hair loss are likely genetically determined [5]. With long-term testosterone use, up to half of transmasculine people will develop androgenic alopecia [15, 31, 40]. Some patients view male-pattern balding as a desirable masculine trait, while others view it as unacceptable. For those patients who seek medical attention for their hair loss, administration of a 5α-reductase inhibitor can be considered [41].

Surveillance (Table 2.2)

Patients undergoing treatment with gender-affirming hormone therapy require regular follow-up to establish the appropriate testosterone dose and assess for any treatment-related adverse effects. While there is no single agreed upon surveillance scheme, both the Endocrine Society and WPATH recommend frequent monitoring at one- to three-month intervals during the first year of treatment, followed by annual or biannual follow-up for stable patients [5, 8]. At each follow-up, blood pressure and weight should be measured [27]. Laboratory studies should be checked, including serum testosterone and estradiol levels, complete blood count, liver enzymes, and a lipid panel. Prior to drawing the serum testosterone level, consideration must be given to the pharmacokinetics of the specific testosterone formulation being used. For those using parenteral testosterone, levels can be checked either midway between injections, or with peaks (24–48 hours after injection) and troughs (immediately before injection) [6]. Pending the results of laboratory studies, testosterone dosage may need to be titrated. The goal is to achieve serum testosterone and estradiol levels in the physiologic male range: 320–1000 ng/dL (10.4–34.7 nmol/L) for testosterone and < 50 pg/mL for estradiol [8].

Risks (Table 2.3)

While gender-affirming hormone therapy is considered safe when prescribed under appropriate medical supervision [6, 29], health risks do exist. These risks should be discussed with patients prior to initiating treatment. Polycythemia, an abnormal elevation of hemoglobin and/or hematocrit, occurs in one in six transgender men receiving testosterone [17]. This condition can occur as a result of the stimulatory effect of testosterone on erythropoiesis [6] and is more likely to occur in patients using intramuscular formulations [73] and/or with supraphysiologic serum testosterone levels [27]. Polycythemia poses a significant health risk, as it increases the risk of venous and arterial thrombosis [42]. When polycythemia is detected, testosterone dosage needs to be decreased, even if serum testosterone levels are within the target range [10].

Additionally, testosterone therapy can worsen metabolic parameters such as triglyceride and low-density lipoprotein levels, BMI, and blood pressure [17, 74, 75]. It has yet to be determined if worsening of these parameters, which are known risk factors for cardiovascular disease, truly increases the risk of cardiovascular disease in transmasculine individuals. While the risk of cardiovascular disease is higher in cisgender men compared with cisgender women, it is unclear if this difference is solely attributable to differences in testosterone levels [27]. The majority of existing research has not demonstrated an increased risk of cardiovascular disease in testosterone-treated transmasculine people [17, 26, 43, 44].

It is also important to consider the potential impact of treatment on bone mineral density (BMD), as testosterone-treated transmasculine people have suppressed estradiol levels. Theoretically, aromatization of androgens to estrogen should

2 Overview of Gender-Affirming Therapy

Table 2.2 Surveillance for patients receiving gender-affirming hormone therapy or puberty suppression [5, 6, 10, 11, 15, 17, 33]

Parameter	Frequency	Goal
Transmasculine		
History	First year: Baseline then every 3 months Following years: 1-2x/year	Patient satisfaction with no side effects
Physical	First year: Baseline then every 3 months Following years: 1-2x/year	Physical masculinization, normal BP, and appropriate weight
Testosterone	First year: Baseline then every 3 months Following years: 1-2x/year	Testosterone level 320–1000 ng/dL
Estradiol	First year: Baseline then every 3 months Following years: 1-2x/year	Estradiol level < 50 pg/mL
CBC	First year: Baseline then every 3 months Following years: 1-2x/year	Hgb and Hct within normal reference range
LFTs	First year: Baseline then every 3 months Following years: 1-2x/year	LFTs within normal reference range
Lipids	Baseline then based on baseline values and CV risk factors	Lipids within normal reference range
Transfeminine		
History	First year: Baseline then every 3 months Following years: 1-2x/year	Patient satisfaction with no side effects
Physical	First year: Baseline then every 3 months Following years: 1-2x/year	Physical feminization, normal BP, and appropriate weight
Testosterone	First year: Baseline then every 3 months Following years: 1-2x/year	Testosterone level < 50 ng/dL
Estradiol	First year: Baseline then every 3 months Following years: 1-2x/year	Estradiol level 100–200 pg/mL
Metabolic profile[a]	First year: Baseline then every 3 months Following years: 1-2x/year	BUN, Cr, and K within normal reference range
Lipids	Not standard practice, at discretion of practitioner	Lipids within normal reference range
Prolactin	Not standard practice, at discretion of practitioner	Prolactin within normal reference range

Note: Abnormal results may warrant more frequent monitoring

Adapted from: Fortin, C.N., Moravek, M.B. Medical Transition for Gender Diverse Patients. *Curr Obstet Gynecol Rep* 9, 166–177 (2020)

BP blood pressure, *BUN* blood urea nitrogen, *CBC* complete blood count, *Cr* creatinine, *CV* cardiovascular, *Hct* hematocrit, *Hgb* hemoglobin, *K* potassium, *LFTs* liver function tests

[a]For patients on spironolactone

Table 2.3 Risks associated with gender-affirming hormone treatment [5, 15, 26, 31, 32, 36, 42–72]

Risk	Masculinizing treatment	Feminizing treatment
Likely increased	Polycythemia Hyperlipidemia Weight gain Hypertension Acne Androgenic alopecia	Venous thromboembolism Weight gain Hyperlipidemia
Possibly increased	Transaminitis Cardiovascular disease Idiopathic intracranial hypertension Sleep apnea	Hyperprolactinemia or prolactinoma Cardiovascular disease Insulin resistance
Not increased	Breast cancer	
Inconclusive	Loss of bone density	Breast cancer Loss of bone density

protect against compromised BMD [45]. In fact, patients who retain their gonads do not appear to have diminished BMD [10, 17, 46]. In a recent cohort study with over 1000 transgender men, the risk of fracture was similar to age-matched cisgender women and lower than age-matched cisgender men [76]. However, there is evidence of compromised BMD in transgender men who have undergone gonadectomy [47].

Although several case reports exist of transgender men developing breast cancer [48, 49, 77], there is currently no evidence of an increased breast cancer risk in transmasculine people receiving gender-affirming hormone therapy [5, 78]. Recently, a large Dutch cohort study demonstrated that the incidence of breast cancer in transgender men was 60-fold higher compared with cisgender men, but five-fold lower compared with cisgender women. For unclear reasons, transgender men diagnosed with breast cancer were significantly younger than cisgender women diagnosed with breast cancer [79]. It has been suggested that the development of breast cancer in these patients is driven by the aromatization of testosterone to estrogen [78]. Alternatively, a mouse model implicated the androgen receptor itself as contributing to breast cancer tumorigenesis [50].

Other possible increased risks amongst transmasculine individuals receiving gender-affirming hormones include transaminitis [29, 30], sleep apnea [5], and idiopathic intracranial hypertension [51, 80]. The long-term health implications of testosterone use have not been well-studied [8, 31].

Surgical Treatment Options

Approximately half of transmasculine individuals on hormone therapy also seek gender-affirming surgery [2]. For many, this is an essential step to alleviate feelings of gender dysphoria. This typically but not always occurs after initiation of hormone therapy [6]. There is no specified order in which surgeries should occur; rather, it is dependent on the individual patient's desires [5]. There are four general criteria per

2 Overview of Gender-Affirming Therapy

the seventh edition of WPATH Standards of Care for undergoing gender-confirming surgery: (1) persistent, well-documented gender dysphoria, (2) capacity to make an informed decision and provide consent, (3) age of majority, and (4) any co-existing medical or mental health concerns are reasonably well-controlled [5] (Table 2.4). Several studies have demonstrated the benefits of gender-affirming surgery, including improvements in well-being and sexual function [52, 53]. Furthermore, the satisfaction rate with gender-affirming surgery is very high [81]. The proportion of individuals who regret having undergone surgery is extremely low (1–2%) [82], even amongst patients who develop surgical complications [5].

Surgical Procedures

Amongst transmasculine patients who opt for gender-confirming surgery, many will choose to solely undergo chest, or "top," surgery [5]. At one institution, as many as 93% of transgender men opting for surgical intervention desired chest surgery [2]. This is typically achieved via subcutaneous mastectomy [7]. Only one referral from a qualified mental health professional is necessary, and hormone therapy is not a prerequisite prior to chest surgery [5]. The overall complication rate is estimated at 12% [83, 84], and can include infection, hematomas or seromas, nipple necrosis, contour irregularities, and scarring [84]. Patients should be counseled preoperatively that they will have a scar when the amount of breast tissue present necessitates skin removal [5].

There are several options for genital surgeries in transmasculine patients including hysterectomy, salpingo-oophorectomy, metoidioplasty or phalloplasty, vaginectomy, scrotoplasty, and implantation of testicular prostheses (Table 2.5) [5]. In one study, 21% of transgender men had undergone hysterectomy and 58% hoped to undergo hysterectomy in the future [1]. Prior to undergoing hysterectomy and/or salpingo-oophorectomy, two referrals are required per WPATH, and the patient should have undergone at least 12 months of continuous hormone therapy, unless medically contraindicated or not clinically indicated for the patient [5, 8]. This

Table 2.4 WPATH criteria for gender-affirming surgeries in adults [5, 10]

Criteria	Chest/breast surgery	Gonadectomy	Genital surgery
# letters required	1	2	2
Persistent, well-documented gender dysphoria	X	X	X
Capacity to make an informed decision and provide consent	X	X	X
Age of majority	X	X	X
Any co-existing medical or mental health concerns are reasonably well-controlled	X	X	X
12 continuous months of hormone therapy [a]		X	X
12 continuous months of living in desired gender role			X

[a]Unless medical contraindication or not clinically indicated

Table 2.5 Options for gender-affirming surgeries [5]

	Masculinizing surgeries	Feminizing surgeries
Breast/chest	Mastectomy	Augmentation mammoplasty
Gonads/genitals	Oophorectomy Hysterectomy Salpingectomy Metoidioplasty Phalloplasty Vaginectomy Scrotoplasty Implantation of testicular prostheses	Orchiectomy Penectomy Orchiectomy Vaginoplasty Clitoroplasty Vulvoplasty
Other	Liposuction/lipofilling Pectoral implants Voice surgery	Facial feminization surgery Waist contouring Voice surgery Reduction thyroid chondroplasty Gluteal augmentation Aesthetic procedures

criterion aims to provide a trial of reversible sex steroid suppression, prior to any irreversible surgical interventions [5]. These criteria also apply to transwomen seeking gonadectomy. The recommended surgical approach is laparoscopic or vaginal, whenever possible. Some patients may opt to undergo vaginectomy at the time of their hysterectomy, although most do not [5].

Metoidioplasty and phalloplasty are the two primary external phallic surgeries available to transmasculine individuals. Phalloplasty is a multistage procedure that involves the creation of a larger phallus, typically via a radial forearm flap [85]. The resultant phallus may allow for penetrative intercourse and standing micturition [86]. During a metoidioplasty, surgeons use the enlarged clitoris to create a one- to three-inch phallus [7]. Ultimately, the vast majority of transmen do not undergo either of these procedures [2, 87], due to lack of access, high cost, and high risk of complications [8]. Although the ultimate cosmetic outcomes for phalloplasty are generally very good, patients should be counseled that achieving standing micturition cannot be guaranteed. Complications associated with the procedure include urinary tract stenosis/fistula and necrosis of the neophallus. As with hysterectomy/salpingo-oophorectomy, per WPATH these surgeries also require two referrals and 12 months of continuous hormone therapy (unless not indicated) [5].

Finally, a number of non-breast, non-genital masculinizing surgeries are also available. These include liposuction, lipofilling, pectoral implants, and voice surgery [5] (Table 2.5).

Perioperative Medication Management

In patients undergoing gender-affirming surgery, it is important to consider how hormone therapies impact perioperative risk. Limited evidence suggests that exogenous testosterone is not associated with increased risk of complications in the

2 Overview of Gender-Affirming Therapy

perioperative period and thus does not need to be discontinued [88]. Following gonadectomy, testosterone therapy needs to be continued indefinitely to maintain masculine secondary sex characteristics, avoid symptoms of hypogonadism, and protect hormone-dependent organ systems [10, 26].

Feminizing Therapies

Hormone Therapies

The typical approach to feminizing hormone therapy involves concurrent administration of estrogen and an anti-androgen [5, 6].

Medications and Regimens (Table 2.1)

The most commonly prescribed estrogen is oral 17-β-estradiol [6]. This agent tends to be preferred due to its ease of use, availability, and relatively low cost [6, 89]. When initiating estrogen therapy, it is recommended to start with a low dose and titrate up as needed to the lowest effective dose. Estradiol tablets can also be taken sublingually. Absorption is significantly increased with sublingual administration, and doses can usually be decreased by half [89]. Oral conjugated estrogens cannot be easily monitored with blood testing and are therefore less frequently utilized as first-line agents [8]. Ethinyl estradiol should also be avoided given its increased thrombogenicity [8]. Transdermal options include an estradiol patch, spray, cream, lotion, or gel [89]. Finally, estradiol valerate and estradiol cypionate, both weekly intramuscular injections, are also available [8].

While adequate testosterone suppression can often be achieved with high doses of estrogen alone, the risks associated with high doses of estrogen are not insignificant. Anti-androgen medications are regularly used in feminizing hormone therapy to reduce the dose of estrogen needed [5]. The most commonly used anti-androgen is spironolactone [5, 8, 40], a potassium-sparing diuretic that binds to the androgen receptor and blocks testosterone secretion [90]. This agent tends to be affordable and widely available [89]. Blood pressure and electrolytes should be regularly monitored, and patients with renal impairment, hepatic disease, or cardiac arrhythmias should avoid this drug due to the risk of hyperkalemia [5, 89]. The 5-α reductase inhibitors, namely finasteride and dutasteride, block conversion of testosterone to the more potent androgen dihydrotestosterone [6]. These drugs have beneficial effects on skin and hair [5]. The two main side effects, gynecomastia and erectile dysfunction, may be viewed positively by many trans women [89]. Androgen receptor blockers are another class of anti-androgens. These agents work by competitively antagonizing the androgen receptor and include bicalutamide and flutamide. Data on the use of these drugs for indications other than the treatment of prostate cancer are scarce. It is important to note that both agents have been associated with hepatotoxicity, and therefore are infrequently used [18, 89].

While not considered first line, suppression of testicular testosterone production can also be achieved by inhibiting pituitary gonadotropin secretion. The two primary agents used for this purpose are GnRH agonists and cyproterone acetate. Cyproterone acetate is an oral progestin that acts by suppressing gonadotropin secretion and antagonizing the androgen receptor [6]. This drug is commonly used in Europe but not approved in the United States due to potential hepatotoxicity [5, 6]. A recent prospective cohort study demonstrated equivalent efficacy in serum testosterone suppression amongst transgender women who received estradiol with either cyproterone acetate or leuprolide acetate [19]. GnRH agonists, although often cost-prohibitive, may be used by patients who cannot tolerate other anti-androgens or do not achieve adequate suppression with estrogen [20, 89]. If used, these agents should be given in conjunction with estradiol to minimize the risk of osteoporosis [91].

The use of progesterone in feminizing hormone therapy is controversial and not considered standard of care [6]. Some providers believe progestin therapy is necessary for full breast development, as progesterone is involved in mammary development in cisgender females [92]. Many patients will request a trial of one of these agents, such as micronized progesterone or medroxyprogesterone acetate, citing anecdotal reports of improved breast development, mood, and libido [21, 93]. However, the use of progestins for this purpose is not recommended by the Endocrine Society [8] as there is very limited evidence of their efficacy in feminizing hormone therapy [30, 54]. Furthermore, progesterone may increase the risk of adverse effects such as venous thromboembolism (VTE), breast cancer, cardiovascular disease, weight gain, and depression [30, 94, 95].

Expected Physical Changes

The earliest effects of feminizing hormone therapy are typically seen within the first few months of treatment and will progress over the course of 2–3 years [8]. Within the first 3 months of treatment, many transfeminine people will experience a decrease in sexual desire and fewer spontaneous erections [8], although most retain the ability to achieve erection and orgasm [89]. The testicles and prostate will eventually atrophy [8].

Changes in body composition can be expected within 3–6 months [6, 8]. Muscle mass and strength decrease, while subcutaneous fat—especially in the hips and thighs—increases [5, 6, 34]. A recent retrospective cohort study found a significant increase in BMI in transgender women after initiation of hormone therapy. This increase occurred primarily in the first 2 years of therapy, followed by a plateau in the third year [38]. Deposition of fat in the face can also occur, which serves to feminize facial features [89]. Height, size of hands and feet, and shape of pelvis will not change if hormone therapy is started after puberty [6]. Breast growth also starts within the first several months of treatment, but maximal development typically takes 2 years [6, 8].

2 Overview of Gender-Affirming Therapy

Changes in hair growth patterns are often the last to occur and can be quite variable. Since the hair growth cycle is a continuous, three- to five-year process involving asynchronous turnover of hair follicles, it takes several years for all existing terminal hairs to be replaced [89]. The only way to accelerate this turnover process is by undergoing electrolysis or laser hair removal [8, 89]. There are limited reports of scalp hair regrowth in transgender women receiving feminizing hormone therapy [22, 96].

Surveillance (Table 2.2)

During the first year of treatment, re-evaluation should occur approximately every 3 months. After the first year, monitoring can be spaced to once or twice a year in stable patients [5, 6, 10]. At each follow-up visit, blood pressure, weight, and relevant laboratory studies should be checked. These include serum testosterone and estradiol levels. Medication dosage should be titrated to achieve levels in the physiologic female range: 100–200 pg/mL for estradiol and < 50 ng/dL for testosterone [6]. It is also important to check a metabolic profile for patients on spironolactone [8]. Some clinicians also monitor estrogen-sensitive laboratory values such as serum prolactin and triglycerides, however this is not considered standard practice [6].

Risks (Table 2.3)

Transfeminine individuals treated with estrogens likely have an increased risk of VTE. This risk is largely dependent on the dose, route, and formulation of estrogen used [97, 98]. As dose increases, so does the risk of VTE [5]. Risk is lower with transdermal administration than with oral administration, likely due to avoidance of the first-pass liver metabolism [8, 95]. Strong consideration should be given to transdermal administration in patients at increased risk for VTE. VTE risk is also increased with concomitant use of third-generation progestins. Patient-specific factors such as obesity, age > 40 years, sedentary lifestyle, and thrombophilic disorders all increase the risk of VTE [5].

Data on cardiovascular risk in estrogen-treated transfeminine individuals are very limited. In a randomized controlled trial, cisgender men given estradiol had a two-fold increase in non-fatal myocardial infarction and cardiovascular deaths compared to the placebo group [55]. There are currently no randomized controlled trials looking at cardiovascular risk in estrogen-treated transfeminine people. Large cohort studies have reported the risk of myocardial infarction in transgender women to be significantly higher than in cisgender women but similar to cisgender men [56, 98]. Estrogen therapy has also been shown to worsen certain metabolic parameters that confer increased cardiovascular disease risk such as hyperlipidemia [93, 99] and insulin resistance [34, 57].

It has been well-established that estrogen induces histologic changes in breast tissue [58] and that hormone therapy use in cisgender postmenopausal women increases breast cancer risk [59, 94, 100]. It is unclear, however, whether this translates into an increased risk of breast cancer in estrogen-treated transgender women. Existing studies have reported conflicting results. While a recent study reported a 46-fold higher risk in transgender women than in cisgender men [79], two older studies suggested a comparable risk to cisgender men [78, 101].

When considering the impact of gender-affirming hormone therapy on BMD, it is important to consider that transgender women have lower BMD than cisgender men prior to starting hormone therapy [17, 60, 102]. Initiating hormone therapy might mitigate this risk, particularly in the short term [61, 76, 103, 104]. Studies on long-term estrogen use have produced mixed results [61, 76, 103, 104]. Available evidence suggests that, amongst patients who do not undergo gonadectomy, hormone therapy does not negatively impact BMD up to 10 years after initiating treatment [46]. The long-term effects of hormone therapy on BMD in transfeminine individuals who do undergo gonadectomy are less clear, with some studies reporting a decrease in BMD and others reporting no change [62, 63, 104]. In one study, low BMD was associated with older age, poorer compliance to hormone therapy, and lower serum estradiol levels [62].

Finally, use of estrogen therapy in transfeminine individuals has been linked to an increased risk of hyperprolactinemia and prolactinoma development in some studies [64–69]. On the other hand, a more recent study showed that the usual treatment regimen with estrogen and spironolactone does not increase serum prolactin levels outside the normal range [70].

Surgical Treatment Options

Surgical Procedures

Transfeminine patients may opt to undergo gender-affirming chest and/or genital surgeries. Chest surgery entails augmentation mammoplasty, with the use of either implants or lipofilling [5]. Patients must have one referral to be eligible for chest surgery. Although not an absolute requirement, both the Endocrine Society and WPATH recommend at least 1–2 years of feminizing hormone therapy prior to breast augmentation in order to maximize breast growth and optimize aesthetic results [5, 8]. The risk of complications in transfeminine individuals undergoing breast augmentation is low but can include infection, seroma, hematoma, and capsular fibrosis [72]. The overall satisfaction rate is high, with one study reporting a 75% long-term satisfaction rate amongst transgender women who underwent implant-based augmentation. The majority of dissatisfaction was attributed to inadequate breast size [105].

Options for feminizing genital surgeries include penectomy, orchiectomy, vaginoplasty, clitoroplasty, and/or vulvoplasty [5] (Table 2.5). Eligibility per WPATH SOC 7 for either orchiectomy or vaginoplasty requires two referrals and 12 months of continuous hormone therapy, unless hormones are medically contraindicated or not clinically indicated for the patient [5, 8]. The most common surgical technique for vaginoplasty is penile skin inversion [5]. With this approach, a vaginal vault is created in the rectourethral space, with a portion of the glans penis used to create the clitoris. After orchiectomy is performed, the scrotal skin is used to create the labia majora. As the scrotal skin contains hair follicles, most surgeons require preoperative hair removal, often via electrolysis, to prevent hair growth in the vagina [7]. Complications are not uncommon and can include delayed healing, neovaginal prolapse, rectovaginal fistula, vaginal or urethral stenosis, and necrosis of the vagina and/or labia [106, 107]. Reported complication rates range from 20 to 49%, with as many as 1/3–1/2 requiring revision surgery [108, 109]. Nevertheless, the overall satisfaction rate amongst transgender women who undergo vaginoplasty has been reported to be as high as 92% [108].

Transfeminine people may also opt for any of a number of non-breast, non-genital surgical interventions. These include facial feminization surgery (which can include facial bone reduction, rhinoplasty, and/or blepharoplasty), contouring of the waist via suction-assisted lipoplasty, voice modification surgery, reduction thyroid chondroplasty (shaving of the Adam's apple), gluteal augmentation with implants or lipofilling [5] (Table 2.5).

Perioperative Medication Management

Given the association between oral estrogens and risk of thromboembolism, many surgeons require discontinuation for several weeks preceding and following surgery [6]. There is insufficient evidence to recommend for or against perioperative discontinuation of transdermal estrogens [88]. A recent study of 178 transgender women undergoing penile inversion vaginoplasty demonstrated no increased risk of VTE amongst patients who continued hormone therapy perioperatively versus those who discontinued 2 weeks preoperatively and 1 week postoperatively. Unfortunately, this study did not specify which routes of estrogen administration were used by patients [71]. Available evidence suggests that spironolactone does not increase the risk of perioperative complications and therefore does not need to be discontinued perioperatively [88]. Postoperatively, hormone therapy regimens often need to be modified if gonadectomy has occurred. Anti-androgen agents should be discontinued, and many providers also decrease estrogen dosage [6].

Management of TGNB Youth

Many TGNB adolescents strongly desire gender-affirming treatment with hormones and surgery. In fact, the number of adolescents who have already socially transitioned to their affirmed gender by the start of high school has continuously increased [5]. The first long-term follow-up study of TGNB youth managed according to clinical practice guidelines (including both gender-affirming hormone therapy and

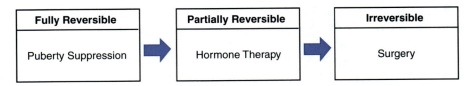

Fig. 2.1 Approach to treatment of transgender adolescents [5]

surgery) demonstrated resolution of gender dysphoria and improvements in psychological functioning. Furthermore, well-being was reported as equal or superior to that of age-matched cisgender young adults. None of the patients regretted undergoing treatment [110]. The management of gender dysphoria in adolescents is complex, as it involves a developmental period marked by significant psychological, physical, and sexual changes. As a result, a different approach than that used in adult patients is required. The management of TGNB youth involves three categories or stages: 1) fully reversible interventions: puberty suppression, 2) partially reversible interventions: hormone therapy, and 3) irreversible interventions: surgical procedures (Fig. 2.1).

Fully Reversible Interventions: Puberty Suppression

There are two main arguments in support of the use of puberty-suppressing agents in TGNB youth. First, it allows adolescents more time to explore their gender identity. Second, preventing the development of secondary sex characteristics may facilitate the adolescent's eventual transition. The recommended treatment duration for puberty suppression is typically a few years, after which the decision is made to either transition to a gender-affirming hormone regimen or discontinue puberty suppression [5].

Prior to initiating puberty suppression, a number of criteria should be met. The adolescent should demonstrate a long-term history of gender dysphoria, which emerged or worsened with the onset of puberty. Any ongoing psychological, social, or medical problems should be addressed prior to treatment initiation. The adolescent must provide informed consent, and if the adolescent has not yet reached the age of consent, consent must be provided by the parents or other caretakers/guardians with assent from the adolescent. Adolescents and their parents should be adequately counseled on the effects of treatment, including the potential impact of treatment on fertility and a discussion on fertility preservation options. Finally, an experienced clinician must agree to the indication for treatment and confirm that puberty has started. It is recommended that at least Tanner Stage 2 is reached, so that adolescents and their parents can make an informed decision about pubertal delay [5, 8].

GnRH agonists, which delay the physical changes of puberty by suppressing estrogen and testosterone production, are the preferred treatment for puberty blocking in adolescents [5, 8]. Leuprolide acetate is given either as an intramuscular injection (monthly or every 3 months) or a subcutaneous injection (monthly or every three, four, or 6 months) [111]. Histrelin is given as a time-release implant that lasts between 12 and 36 months [7]. There is currently insufficient evidence to support the use of one monitoring scheme in adolescents treated with GnRH agonists over another [7, 8, 112]. The Endocrine Society recommends initially assessing height, weight, blood pressure, and Tanner stages every 3–6 months, as well as laboratory studies (luteinizing hormone, follicle stimulating hormone, estradiol, testosterone, vitamin D) every six to 12 months [8]. Others also recommend checking additional laboratory studies such as renal and liver function, lipids, glucose, insulin, and glycosylated hemoglobin annually [7]. Bone density should be assessed via dual-energy X-ray absorptiometry (DXA) every 1–2 years [8].

GnRH agonists are overall well-tolerated. In one study of 27 transgender youth undergoing puberty suppression with GnRH agonists, only one patient discontinued treatment, citing emotional lability [113]. Other bothersome side effects can include hot flashes and fatigue [8]. These agents are also overall considered to be safe. The primary safety concern is the potential negative impact on BMD, as bone mineralization relies on sex steroids [114–117]. Bone mass does not increase, but typically is not lost, throughout the duration of administration [118]. For this reason, it is recommended that the treatment duration does not exceed a few years [7]. Concerns have also been raised about the impact of these agents on brain development [8]. Animal studies have demonstrated effects on spatial memory, social behavior, and stress regulation [119–121]. As of yet, no evidence of compromised executive function has been identified in humans [122]. Finally, recent evidence indicates that treatment with GnRH agonists in transgender youth may increase diastolic blood pressure [123].

The primary disadvantage of GnRH agonists for many patients is their cost. If cost-prohibitive, alternative agents can be considered. Progestins, most commonly medroxyprogesterone, can be used to suppress menses in transmasculine patients [5]. Unfortunately, these agents are not as effective as GnRH agonists at decreasing endogenous sex hormones and can also be associated with other side effects [124]. Continuous oral contraceptives can also be used to achieve menstrual suppression. In transfeminine patients, anti-androgens such as spironolactone can be used to decrease the effects of endogenous androgens [5].

Partially Reversible Interventions: Hormone Therapy

Feminizing or masculinizing hormones can be initiated in adolescents after the persistence of gender dysphoria has been confirmed by medical and mental health professionals. Furthermore, the adolescent must have sufficient mental capacity to provide informed consent, which most adolescents reach by age 16. There are very few studies which have reported the use of gender-affirming hormone therapy in adolescents under the age of 14 [8]. Ideally, parental consent will also be provided prior to hormone initiation. Patients should be counseled that not all hormone-induced physical changes will be reversible. Some changes, such as estrogen-induced gynecomastia, may require reconstructive surgery for reversal, whereas other changes, like deepening of the voice induced by testosterone, are irreversible [5]. It is recommended that treatment is initiated with a gradually increasing dose schedule [8].

Similar to the recommended monitoring scheme in adolescents undergoing puberty suppression, the Endocrine Society recommends assessing height, weight, blood pressure, and Tanner stage every 3–6 months in adolescents receiving hormone therapy. In transmasculine youth, hemoglobin/hematocrit, lipids, testosterone, and vitamin D levels should be checked every six to 12 months, whereas prolactin, estradiol, and vitamin D levels should be checked at the same interval in transfeminine youth. BMD should be assessed using DXA every 1–2 years. BMD screening should continue into adulthood, typically until age 25–30 years or until peak bone mass has been reached [8].

Irreversible Interventions: Surgery

In order for a transgender adolescent to be eligible for genital surgery, the following criteria must be met: (1) the patient has reached the legal age of majority to provide consent to medical procedures.

Conclusion

Gender-affirming treatment incorporates hormone therapy and surgical intervention. Hormone therapy is overall safe and effective for most TGNB individuals. It is important to regularly monitor for adverse effects and risks associated with hormone use. Many patients will also opt for surgical intervention(s), which can include chest surgeries, gonadectomy, genital surgeries, and a variety of other masculinizing/feminizing procedures. High-quality prospective studies are necessary to improve our understanding of long-term outcomes for patients receiving gender-affirming treatment.

References

1. Grant JM, Mottet LA, Tanis J, Herman JL, Harrison J, Keisling M. National transgender discrimination survey report on health and health care [internet]. Washington D.C.: 2010.
2. Kailas M, Lu HMS, Rothman EF, Safer JD. Prevalence and types of gender-affirming surgery among a sample of transgender endocrinology patients prior to state expansion of insurance coverage. Endocr Pract. 2017;23(7):780–6.

3. James SE, Herman JL, Rankin S, Keisling M, Mottet L, Anafi M. The Report of the 2015 U.S. Washington, DC: Transgender Survey; 2016.
4. Leinung M, Urizar M, Patel N, Sood S. Endocrine treatment of transsexual persons: extensive personal experience. Endocr Pract. 2013;19(4):644–50.
5. Coleman E, Bockting W, Botzer M, Cohen-Kettenis P, DeCuypere G, Feldman J, et al. Standards of care for the health of transsexual, trans-gender, and gender-nonconforming people, version 7. Int J Transgenderism. 2012;13(4):165.
6. Safer JD, Tangpricha V. Care of the transgender patient. Ann Intern Med. 2019;171(1): ITC1–14.
7. Center of Excellence for Transgender Health. Guidelines for the primary and gender-affirming Care of Transgender and Gender Nonbinary People. San Fr: Univ California; 2016.
8. Hembree WC, Cohen-Kettenis PT, Gooren L, Hannema SE, Meyer WJ, Murad MH, et al. Endocrine treatment of gender-dysphoric/gender-incongruent persons: an Endocrine Society clinical practice guideline. J Clin Endocrinol Metab. 2017;102(11):3869–903.
9. Pelusi C, Costantino A, Martelli V, Lambertini M, Bazzocchi A, Ponti F, et al. Effects of three different testosterone formulations in female-to-male transsexual persons. J Sex Med. 2014;11(12):3002–11.
10. Meriggiola MC, Gava G. Endocrine care of transpeople part I. a review of cross-sex hormonal treatments, outcomes and adverse effects in transmen. Clin Endocrinol. 2015;83(5):597–606.
11. McFarland J, Craig W, Clarke NJ, Spratt DI. Serum testosterone concentrations remain stable between injections in patients receiving subcutaneous testosterone. J Endocr Soc. 2017;1(8):1095–103.
12. Spratt DI, Stewart II, Savage C, Craig W, Spack NP, Chandler DW, et al. Subcutaneous injection of testosterone is an effective and preferred alternative to intramuscular injection: demonstration in female-to-male transgender patients. J Clin Endocrinol Metab. 2017;102(7):2349–55.
13. Mueller A, Kiesewetter F, Binder H, Beckmann MW, Dittrich R. Long-term administration of testosterone undecanoate every 3 months for testosterone supplementation in female-to-male transsexuals. J Clin Endocrinol Metab. 2007;92(9):3470–5.
14. Asscheman H, Gooren LJG, Eklund PLE. Mortality and morbidity in transsexual patients with cross-gender hormone treatment. Metabolism. 1989;38(9):869–73.
15. Gooren LJG, Giltay EJ. Review of studies of androgen treatment of female-to-male transsexuals: effects and risks of administration of androgens to females. J Sex Med. 2008;5(4):765–76.
16. Cosyns M, Van Borsel J, Wierckx K, Dedecker D, Van De Peer F, Daelman T, et al. Voice in female-to-male transsexual persons after long-term androgen therapy. Laryngoscope. 2014;124(6):1409–14.
17. Wierckx K, Mueller S, Weyers S, Van Caenegem E, Roef G, Heylens G, et al. Long-term evaluation of cross-sex hormone treatment in transsexual persons. J Sex Med. 2012;9(10):2641–51.
18. Kolvenbag GJCM, Blackledge GRP. Worldwide activity and safety of bicalutamide: a summary review. Urology. 1996;47(1 SUPPL. 1):70–9.
19. Gava G, Mancini I, Alvisi S, Seracchioli R, Meriggiola MC. A comparison of 5-year administration of cyproterone acetate or leuprolide acetate in combination with estradiol in transwomen. Eur J Endocrinol. 2020;163(6):561–9.
20. Pappas II, Craig WY, Spratt LV, Spratt DI. Efficacy of sex steroid therapy without progestin or GnRH agonist for gonadal suppression in adult transgender patients. J Clin Endocrinol Metab. 2020;106(3):e1290–300.
21. Jain J, Kwan D, Forcier M. Medroxyprogesterone acetate in gender-affirming therapy for transwomen: results from a retrospective study. J Clin Endocrinol Metab. 2019;104(11):5148–56.
22. Adenuga P, Summers P, Bergfeld W. Hair regrowth in a male patient with extensive androgenetic alopecia on estrogen therapy. J Am Acad Dermatol. 2012;67(3):e121.
23. Jockenhövel F. Testosterone therapy - what, when and to whom? Aging Male. 2004;7(4):319–24.

24. Turner L, Ly LP, Desai R, Singh GKS, Handelsman TD, Savkovic S, et al. Pharmacokinetics and acceptability of subcutaneous injection of testosterone undecanoate. J Endocr Soc. 2019;3(8):1531–40.
25. Swerdloff RS, Wang C, White WB, Kaminetsky J, Gittelman MC, Longstreth JA, et al. A new oral testosterone undecanoate formulation restores testosterone to normal concentrations in hypogonadal men. J Clin Endocrinol Metab. 2020;105(8):2515.
26. Gooren LJ. Care of transsexual persons. N Engl J Med. 2011;364(13):1251–7.
27. Moravek MB. Gender-affirming hormone therapy for transgender men. Clin Obstet Gynecol. 2018;61(4):687–704.
28. Cler GJ, McKenna VS, Dahl KL, Stepp CE. Longitudinal case study of transgender voice changes under testosterone hormone therapy. J Voice. 2020;34(5):748–62.
29. Wierckx K, Van Caenegem E, Schreiner T, Haraldsen I, Fisher A, Toye K, et al. Cross-sex hormone therapy in trans persons is safe and effective at short-time follow-up: results from the European network for the investigation of gender incongruence. J Sex Med. 2014;11(8):1999–2011.
30. Meyer WJ, Webb A, Stuart CA, Finkelstein JW, Lawrence B, Walker PA. Physical and hormonal evaluation of transsexual patients: a longitudinal study. Arch Sex Behav. 1986;15(2):121–38.
31. Irwig MS. Testosterone therapy for transgender men. Lancet Diabetes Endocrinol. 2017;5(4):301–11.
32. Gooren LJ, Giltay EJ, Bunck MC. Long-term treatment of transsexuals with cross-sex hormones: extensive personal experience. J Clin Endocrinol Metab. 2008;93(1):19–25.
33. Wiik A, Lundberg TR, Rullman E, Andersson DP, Holmberg M, Mandić M, et al. Muscle strength, size, and composition following 12 months of gender-affirming treatment in transgender individuals. J Clin Endocrinol Metab. 2020;105(3):e805.
34. Shadid S, Abosi-Appeadu K, De Maertelaere AS, Defreyne J, Veldeman L, Holst JJ, et al. Effects of gender-affirming hormone therapy on insulin sensitivity and incretin responses in transgender people. Diabetes Care. 2020;43(2):411–7.
35. Klaver M, Dekker MJHJ, de Mutsert R, Twisk JWR, den Heijer M. Cross-sex hormone therapy in transgender persons affects total body weight, body fat and lean body mass: a meta-analysis. Andrologia. 2017;49(5):e12660.
36. Deutsch MB, Bhakri V, Kubicek K. Effects of cross-sex hormone treatment on transgender women and men. Obstet Gynecol. 2015;125(3):605–10.
37. Sequeira GM, Kidd K, El Nokali NE, Rothenberger SD, Levine MD, Montano GT, et al. Early effects of testosterone initiation on body mass index in transmasculine adolescents. J Adolesc Health. 2019;65(6):818–20.
38. Suppakitjanusant P, Ji Y, Stevenson MO, Chantrapanichkul P, Sineath RC, Goodman M, et al. Effects of gender affirming hormone therapy on body mass index in transgender individuals: a longitudinal cohort study. J Clin Transl Endocrinol. 2020;21:100230.
39. Olson-Kennedy J, Okonta V, Clark LF, Belzer M. Physiologic response to gender-affirming hormones among transgender youth. J Adolesc Health. 2018;62(4):397–401.
40. Marks DH, Hagigeorges D, Manatis-Lornell AJ, Dommasch E, Senna MM. Hair loss among transgender and gender-nonbinary patients: a cross-sectional study. Br J Dermatol. 2019;181(5):1082–3.
41. Irwig MS. Safety concerns regarding 5α reductase inhibitors for the treatment of androgenetic alopecia. Curr Opin Endocrinol Diabetes Obes. 2015;22(3):248–53.
42. Byrnes JR, Wolberg AS. Red blood cells in thrombosis. Blood. 2017;130(16):1795–9.
43. Asscheman H, Giltay EJ, Megens JAJ, De Ronde W, Van Trotsenburg MAA, Gooren LJG. A long-term follow-up study of mortality in transsexuals receiving treatment with cross-sex hormones. Eur J Endocrinol. 2011;164(4):635–42.
44. Streed CG, Harfouch O, Marvel F, Blumenthal RS, Martin SS, Mukherjee M. Cardiovascular disease among transgender adults receiving hormone therapy: a narrative review. Ann Intern Med. 2017;167(4):256–67.

2 Overview of Gender-Affirming Therapy

45. Lips P, van Kesteren PJM, Asscheman H, Gooren LJG. The effect of androgen treatment on bone metabolism in female-to-male transsexuals. J Bone Miner Res. 2009;11(11):1769–73.
46. Wiepjes CM, de Jongh RT, de Blok CJM, Vlot MC, Lips P, Twisk JWR, et al. Bone safety during the first ten years of gender-affirming hormonal treatment in transwomen and transmen. J Bone Miner Res. 2019;34(3):447–54.
47. Dobrolińska M, van der Tuuk K, Vink P, van den Berg M, Schuringa A, Monroy-Gonzalez AG, et al. Bone mineral density in transgender individuals after gonadectomy and long-term gender-affirming hormonal treatment. J Sex Med. 2019;16(9):1469–77.
48. Burcombe RJ, Makris A, Pittam M, Finer N. Breast cancer after bilateral subcutaneous mastectomy in a female-to-male trans-sexual. Breast. 2003;12(4):290–3.
49. Shao T, Grossbard ML, Klein P. Breast cancer in female-to-male transsexuals: two cases with a review of physiology and management. Clin Breast Cancer. 2011;11(6):417–9.
50. Feng J, Li L, Zhang N, Liu J, Zhang L, Gao H, et al. Androgen and AR contribute to breast cancer development and metastasis: an insight of mechanisms. Oncogene. 2017;36(20):2775–90.
51. Park S, Cheng CP, Lim LT, Gerber D. Secondary intracranial hypertension from testosterone therapy in a transgender patient. Semin Ophthalmol. 2014;29(3):156–8.
52. De Cuypere G, T'Sjoen G, Beerten R, Selvaggi G, De Sutter P, Hoebeke P, et al. Sexual and physical health after sex reassignment surgery. Arch Sex Behav. 2005;34(6):679–90.
53. Klein C, Gorzalka BB. Sexual functioning in transsexuals following hormone therapy and genital surgery: a review. J Sex Med. 2009;6(11):2922–39.
54. Wierckx K, Gooren L, T'Sjoen G. Clinical review: breast development in trans women receiving cross-sex hormones. J Sex Med. 2014;11(5):1240–7.
55. The Coronary Drug Project. Initial findings leading to modifications of its research protocol. JAMA. 1970;214(7):1303–13.
56. Alzahrani T, Nguyen T, Ryan A, Dwairy A, McCaffrey J, Yunus R, et al. Cardiovascular disease risk factors and myocardial infarction in the transgender population. Circ Cardiovasc Qual Outcomes. 2019;12(4):e005597.
57. Spanos C, Bretherton I, Zajac JD, Cheung AS. Effects of gender-affirming hormone therapy on insulin resistance and body composition in transgender individuals: a systematic review. World J Diabetes. 2020;11(3):66–77.
58. Grynberg M, Fanchin R, Dubost G, Colau JC, Brémont-Weil C, Frydman R, et al. Histology of genital tract and breast tissue after long-term testosterone administration in a female-to-male transsexual population. Reprod Biomed Online. 2010;20(4):553–8.
59. Banks E, Beral V, Bull D, Reeves G, Austoker J, English R, et al. Breast cancer and hormone-replacement therapy in the million women study. Lancet. 2003;362(9382):419–27.
60. Van Caenegem E, Taes Y, Wierckx K, Vandewalle S, Toye K, Kaufman JM, et al. Low bone mass is prevalent in male-to-female transsexual persons before the start of cross-sex hormonal therapy and gonadectomy. Bone. 2013;54(1):92–7.
61. Sosa M, Jódar E, Arbelo E, Domínguez C, Saavedra P, Torres A, et al. Bone mass, bone turnover, vitamin D, and estrogen receptor gene polymorphisms in male to female transsexuals: effects of estrogenic treatment on bone metabolism of the male. J Clin Densitom. 2003;6(3):297–304.
62. Motta G, Marinelli L, Barale M, Brustio PR, Manieri C, Ghigo E, et al. Fracture risk assessment in an Italian group of transgender women after gender-confirming surgery. J Bone Miner Metab. 2020;38(6):885.
63. T'Sjoen G, Weyers S, Taes Y, Lapauw B, Toye K, Goemaere S, et al. Prevalence of low bone mass in relation to estrogen treatment and body composition in male-to-female transsexual persons. J Clin Densitom. 2009;12(3):306–13.
64. Nota NM, Dekker MJHJ, Klaver M, Wiepjes CM, van Trotsenburg MA, Heijboer AC, et al. Prolactin levels during short- and long-term cross-sex hormone treatment: an observational study in transgender persons. Andrologia. 2017;49(6):e12666.
65. Bunck MC, Debono M, Giltay EJ, Verheijen AT, Diamant M, Gooren LJ. Autonomous prolactin secretion in two male-to-female transgender patients using conventional oestrogen dosages. BMJ Case Rep. 2009;2009:bcr0220091589.

66. Cunha FS, Domenice S, Câmara VL, Sircili MHP, Gooren LJG, Mendonça BB, et al. Diagnosis of prolactinoma in two male-to-female transsexual subjects following high-dose cross-sex hormone therapy. Andrologia. 2015;47(6):680–4.
67. Kovacs K, Stefaneanu L, Ezzat S, Smyth HS. Prolactin-producing pituitary adenoma in a male-to-female transsexual patient with protracted estrogen administration: a morphologic study. Arch Pathol Lab Med. 1994;118(5):562–5.
68. Asscheman H, Gooren LJG, Assies J, Smits JPH, De Slegte R. Prolactin levels and pituitary enlargement in hormone-treated male-to-female transsexuals. Clin Endocrinol. 1988;28(6):583–8.
69. Serri O, Noiseux D, Robert F, Hardy J. Lactotroph hyperplasia in an estrogen treated male-to-female transsexual patient. J Clin Endocrinol Metab. 1996;81(9):3177–9.
70. Bisson JR, Chan KJ, Safer JD. Prolactin levels do not rise among transgender women treated with estradiol and spironolactone. Endocr Pract. 2018;24(7):646–51.
71. Nolan IT, Haley C, Morrison SD, Pannucci CJ, Satterwhite T. Estrogen continuation and venous thromboembolism in penile inversion vaginoplasty. J Sex Med. 2020;18(1):193–200.
72. Kanhai RCJ, Hage JJ, Karim RB, Mulder JW. Exceptional presenting conditions and outcome of augmentation mammaplasty in male-to-female transsexuals. Ann Plast Surg. 1999;43(5):476–83.
73. Nolan BJ, Leemaqz SY, Ooi O, Cundill P, Silberstein N, Locke P, et al. Prevalence of polycythaemia with different formulations of testosterone therapy in transmasculine individuals. Intern Med J. 2020;51(6):873–8.
74. Weinand JD, Safer JD. Hormone therapy in transgender adults is safe with provider supervision; a review of hormone therapy sequelae for transgender individuals. J Clin Transl Endocrinol. 2015;2(2):55–60.
75. Elamin MB, Garcia MZ, Murad MH, Erwin PJ, Montori VM. Effect of sex steroid use on cardiovascular risk in transsexual individuals: a systematic review and meta-analyses. Clin Endocrinol. 2010;72(1):1–10.
76. Wiepjes CM, de Blok CJM, Staphorsius AS, Nota NM, Vlot MC, de Jongh RT, et al. Fracture risk in trans women and trans men using long-term gender-affirming hormonal treatment: a nationwide cohort study. J Bone Miner Res. 2020;35(1):64–70.
77. Nikolic DV, Djordjevic ML, Granic M, Nikolic AT, Stanimirovic VV, Zdravkovic D, et al. Importance of revealing a rare case of breast cancer in a female to male transsexual after bilateral mastectomy. World J Surg Oncol. 2012;10:280.
78. Gooren LJ, van Trotsenburg MAAA, Giltay EJ, van Diest PJ. Breast cancer development in transsexual subjects receiving cross-sex hormone treatment. J Sex Med. 2013;10(12):3129–34.
79. De Blok CJM, Wiepjes CM, Nota NM, Van Engelen K, Adank MA, Dreijerink KMA, et al. Breast cancer risk in transgender people receiving hormone treatment: Nationwide cohort study in the Netherlands. BMJ. 2019;365:l1652.
80. Nguyen HV, Gilbert AL, Fortin E, Vodopivec I, Torun N, Chwalisz BK, et al. Elevated intracranial pressure associated with exogenous hormonal therapy used for gender affirmation. J Neuro-Ophthalmol. 2020;41(2):217–23.
81. Murad MH, Elamin MB, Garcia MZ, Mullan RJ, Murad A, Erwin PJ, et al. Hormonal therapy and sex reassignment: a systematic review and meta-analysis of quality of life and psychosocial outcomes. Clin Endocrinol. 2010;72(2):214–31.
82. Lawrence AA. Patient-reported complications and functional outcomes of male-to-female sex reassignment surgery. Arch Sex Behav. 2006;35(6):717–27.
83. Wolter A, Diedrichson J, Scholz T, Arens-Landwehr A, Liebau J. Sexual reassignment surgery in female-to-male transsexuals: an algorithm for subcutaneous mastectomy. J Plast Reconstr Aesthetic Surg. 2015;68(2):184–91.
84. Monstrey S, Selvaggi G, Ceulemans P, Van Landuyt K, Bowman C, Blondeel P, et al. Chest-wall contouring surgery in female-to-male transsexuals: a new algorithm. Plast Reconstr Surg. 2008;121(3):849–59.

2 Overview of Gender-Affirming Therapy

85. Wroblewski P, Gustafsson J, Selvaggi G. Sex reassignment surgery for transsexuals. Curr Opin Endocrinol Diabetes Obes. 2013;20(6):570–4.
86. Nolan IT, Kuhner CJ, Dy GW. Demographic and temporal trends in transgender identities and gender confirming surgery. Transl Androl Urol. 2019;8(3):184–90.
87. Beckwith N, Reisner SL, Zaslow S, Mayer KH, Keuroghlian AS. Factors associated with gender-affirming surgery and age of hormone therapy initiation among transgender adults. Transgender Heal. 2017;2(1):156–64.
88. Boskey ER, Taghinia AH, Ganor O. Association of surgical risk with exogenous hormone use in transgender patients: a systematic review. JAMA Surg. 2019;154(2):109–15.
89. Randolph JF. Gender-affirming hormone therapy for transgender females. Clin Obstet Gynecol. 2018;61(4):705–21.
90. Prior JC, Vigna YM, Watson D. Spironolactone with physiological female steroids for presurgical therapy of male-to-female transsexualism. Arch Sex Behav. 1989;18(1):49–57.
91. Prince JCJ, Safer JD. Endocrine treatment of transgender individuals: current guidelines and strategies. Expert Rev Endocrinol Metab. 2020;15(6):395–403.
92. Oriel KA. Medical care of transsexual patients. J Gay Lesbian Med Assoc. 2000;4(4):185–94.
93. Dutra E, Lee J, Torbati T, Garcia M, Merz CNB, Shufelt C. Cardiovascular implications of gender-affirming hormone treatment in the transgender population. Maturitas. 2019;129:45–9.
94. Rossouw JE, Anderson GL, Prentice RL, LaCroix AZ, Kooperberg C, Stefanick ML, et al. Risks and benefits of estrogen plus progestin in healthy postmenopausal women: principal results from the women's health initiative randomized controlled trial. J Am Med Assoc. 2002;288(3):321–33.
95. Vinogradova Y, Coupland C, Hippisley-Cox J. Use of hormone replacement therapy and risk of venous thromboembolism: Nested case-control studies using the QResearch and CPRD databases. BMJ. 2019;364:k4810.
96. Stevenson MO, Wixon N, Safer JD. Scalp hair regrowth in hormone-treated transgender women. Transgender Heal. 2016;1(1):202–4.
97. Nota NM, Wiepjes CM, De Blok CJM, Gooren LJG, Kreukels BPC, Den Heijer M. Occurrence of acute cardiovascular events in transgender individuals receiving hormone therapy. Circulation. 2019;139(11):1461–2.
98. Getahun D, Nash R, Flanders WD, Baird TC, Becerra-Culqui TA, Cromwell L, et al. Cross-sex hormones and acute cardiovascular events in transgender persons: a cohort study. Ann Intern Med. 2018;169(4):205–13.
99. Maraka S, Ospina NS, Rodriguez-Gutierrez R, Davidge-Pitts CJ, Nippoldt TB, Prokop LJ, et al. Sex steroids and cardiovascular outcomes in transgender individuals: a systematic review and meta-analysis. J Clin Endocrinol Metab. 2017;102(11):3914–23.
100. Colditz GA, Hankinson SE, Hunter DJ, Willett WC, Manson JE, Stampfer MJ, et al. The use of estrogens and progestins and the risk of breast cancer in postmenopausal women. N Engl J Med. 1995;332(24):1589–93.
101. Brown GR, Jones KT. Incidence of breast cancer in a cohort of 5,135 transgender veterans. Breast Cancer Res Treat. 2015;149(1):191–8.
102. Stevenson MO, Tangpricha V. Osteoporosis and bone health in transgender persons. Endocrinol Metab Clin N Am. 2019;48(2):421–7.
103. Ruetsche AG, Kneubuehl R, Birkhaeuser MH, Lippuner K. Cortical and trabecular bone mineral density in transsexuals after long-term cross-sex hormonal treatment: a cross-sectional study. Osteoporos Int. 2005;16(7):791–8.
104. Lapauw B, Taes Y, Simoens S, Van Caenegem E, Weyers S, Goemaere S, et al. Body composition, volumetric and areal bone parameters in male-to-female transsexual persons. Bone. 2008;43(6):1016–21.
105. Kanhai RCJ, Hage JJ, Mulder JW. Long-term outcome of augmentation mammaplasty in male-to-female transsexuals: a questionnaire survey of 107 patients. Br J Plast Surg. 2000;53(3):209–11.

106. Bucci S, Mazzon G, Liguori G, Napoli R, Pavan N, Bormioli S, et al. Neovaginal prolapse in male-to-female transsexuals: an 18-year-long experience. Biomed Res Int. 2014;2014:1.
107. Raigosa M, Avvedimento S, Yoon TS, Cruz-Gimeno J, Rodriguez G, Fontdevila J. Male-to-female genital reassignment surgery: a retrospective review of surgical technique and complications in 60 patients. J Sex Med. 2015;12(8):1837–45.
108. Loree JT, Loree JT, Burke MS, Rippe B, Clarke S, Moore SH, et al. Transfeminine gender confirmation surgery with penile inversion vaginoplasty: an initial experience. Plast Reconstr Surg - Glob Open. 2020;8(5):e2873.
109. Ferrando CA. Adverse events associated with gender affirming vaginoplasty surgery. Am J Obstet Gynecol. 2020;223(2):267.e1–6.
110. De Vries ALC, McGuire JK, Steensma TD, Wagenaar ECF, Doreleijers TAH, Cohen-Kettenis PT. Young adult psychological outcome after puberty suppression and gender reassignment. Pediatrics. 2014;134(4):696–704.
111. Rosenthal SM. Approach to the patient: transgender youth: endocrine considerations. J Clin Endocrinol Metab. 2014;99(12):4379–89.
112. Carel JC, Eugster EA, Rogol A, Ghizzoni L, Palmert MR. Consensus statement on the use of gonadotropin-releasing hormone analogs in children. Pediatrics. 2009;123(4):e752.
113. Khatchadourian K, Amed S, Metzger DL. Clinical management of youth with gender dysphoria in Vancouver. J Pediatr. 2014;164(4):906–11.
114. Klink D, Caris M, Heijboer A, Van Trotsenburg M, Rotteveel J. Bone mass in young adulthood following gonadotropin-releasing hormone analog treatment and cross-sex hormone treatment in adolescents with gender dysphoria. J Clin Endocrinol Metab. 2015;100(2):E270–5.
115. Vlot MC, Klink DT, den Heijer M, Blankenstein MA, Rotteveel J, Heijboer AC. Effect of pubertal suppression and cross-sex hormone therapy on bone turnover markers and bone mineral apparent density (BMAD) in transgender adolescents. Bone. 2017;95:11–9.
116. Joseph T, Ting J, Butler G. The effect of GnRH analogue treatment on bone mineral density in young adolescents with gender dysphoria: findings from a large national cohort. J Pediatr Endocrinol Metab. 2019;32(10):1077.
117. Stoffers IE, de Vries MC, Hannema SE. Physical changes, laboratory parameters, and bone mineral density during testosterone treatment in adolescents with gender dysphoria. J Sex Med. 2019;16(9):1459–68.
118. Delemarre-Van De Waal HA, Cohen-Kettenis PT. Clinical management of gender identity disorder in adolescents: a protocol on psychological and paediatric endocrinology aspects. Eur J Endocrinol Suppl. 2006;155(1):S131–7.
119. Anacker C, Sydnor E, Chen BK, LaGamma CC, McGowan JC, Mastrodonato A, et al. Behavioral and neurobiological effects of GnRH agonist treatment in mice—potential implications for puberty suppression in transgender individuals. Neuropsychopharmacology. 2020;46:882–90.
120. Hough D, Bellingham M, Haraldsen IRH, McLaughlin M, Rennie M, Robinson JE, et al. Spatial memory is impaired by peripubertal GnRH agonist treatment and testosterone replacement in sheep. Psychoneuroendocrinology. 2017;75:173–82.
121. Wojniusz S, Vögele C, Ropstad E, Evans N, Robinson J, Sütterlin S, et al. Prepubertal gonadotropin-releasing hormone analog leads to exaggerated behavioral and emotional sex differences in sheep. Horm Behav. 2011;59(1):22–7.
122. Staphorsius AS, Kreukels BPC, Cohen-Kettenis PT, Veltman DJ, Burke SM, Schagen SEE, et al. Puberty suppression and executive functioning: an fMRI-study in adolescents with gender dysphoria. Psychoneuroendocrinology. 2015;56:190–9.
123. Perl L, Segev-Becker A, Israeli G, Elkon-Tamir E, Oren A. Blood pressure dynamics after pubertal suppression with gonadotropin-releasing hormone analogs followed by testosterone treatment in transgender male adolescents: a pilot study. LGBT Heal. 2020;7(6):340–4.
124. Lynch MM, Khandheria MM, Meyer WJ. Retrospective study of the management of childhood and adolescent gender identity disorder using medroxyprogesterone acetate. Int J Transgenderism. 2015;16(4):201–8.

Chapter 3
Effects of Masculinizing Therapy on Reproductive Capacity

Hadrian M. Kinnear and Molly B. Moravek

Introduction

Many transgender and non-binary (TGNB) people pursue gender-affirming hormone therapy and/or surgeries to develop physical characteristics of their affirmed gender. In general, transgender men or transmasculine individuals were assigned female and may seek gender-affirming post pubertal hormonal therapy in the form of testosterone. Testosterone is administered via intramuscular or subcutaneous injections or via a transdermal gel or patch and is often continued indefinitely depending on patient goals and needs. Clinicians may monitor testosterone levels to ensure they are within the normal range for cisgender (non-transgender) men [1], again depending on the goals of the individual as some patients may be on a low or microdose protocol. Masculinizing effects of testosterone often include voice deepening, cessation of menses, clitoral enlargement, body fat redistribution, and growth of body hair [2].

Transmasculine patients are prescribed testosterone without a concrete understanding of the impact of this often long-term therapy on their reproductive health. National and international medical organizations recommend counseling about

H. M. Kinnear (✉)
Program in Cellular and Molecular Biology, University of Michigan, Ann Arbor, MI, USA

Medical Scientist Training Program, University of Michigan, Ann Arbor, MI, USA
e-mail: hkinnear@med.umich.edu

M. B. Moravek
Division of Reproductive Endocrinology and Infertility, University of Michigan, Ann Arbor, MI, USA

Department of Obstetrics and Gynecology, University of Michigan, Ann Arbor, MI, USA

Department of Urology, University of Michigan, Ann Arbor, MI, USA
e-mail: mpenderg@med.umich.edu

© The Author(s), under exclusive license to Springer Nature Switzerland AG 2023
M. B. Moravek, G. de Haan (eds.), *Reproduction in Transgender and Nonbinary Individuals*, https://doi.org/10.1007/978-3-031-14933-7_3

fertility preservation prior to starting gender-affirming hormones [1–3]; however, these recommendations reflect an assumption of testosterone-induced fertility loss based on conflicting and limited data. Transmasculine fertility preservation can be challenging, as oocyte or embryo cryopreservation is expensive, invasive, and time-consuming. Due to these hurdles, many transmasculine individuals do not undergo fertility preservation prior to starting testosterone but later may be interested in using their gametes for reproduction or being a gestational parent [4, 5]. Although there are limited data on fertility following gender-affirming testosterone, there has been a recent increase in research attention in this area. Encouragingly, studies suggest that reproductive potential may remain after testosterone therapy for at least some individuals [6–10]. Hopefully additional research will lead to future clinical guidelines that offer more nuanced perspectives regarding reproductive options after prolonged testosterone.

In this chapter, we review what is currently known regarding the impact of masculinizing testosterone on the reproductive tract (ovaries, uterus, fallopian tubes) and describe emerging data regarding pregnancy and assisted reproductive technologies (ART). We then discuss relevant animal models and highlight key unanswered questions.

Impact of Testosterone on the Ovaries

Although ovaries from individuals treated with testosterone appear to share multiple characteristics with polycystic ovary morphology, these similarities do not necessarily imply broad associations between testosterone therapy and the multifactorial and complex polycystic ovary syndrome (PCOS). Multiple studies have noted increased tunica albuginea or outer cortex collagenization, stromal hyperplasia, and stromal luteinization in testosterone-exposed ovaries (Table 3.1). These characteristics are also frequently observed in PCOS [22]. Ovarian follicular changes with testosterone therapy have also been observed, although studies differ with regard to their definitions and terminology. Studies of testosterone-exposed ovaries from transgender men have reported multifollicular ovaries, multiple cystic follicles, antral follicle counts of greater than 12 follicles in an ovary, or similar follicle counts with increased atretic follicles (Table 3.1). Variable terminology and classifications have led to apparent conflict, with some studies reporting testosterone leads to polycystic ovary morphology [12, 14, 15, 17] and others disagreeing [18, 23]. Most studies of ovarian histopathology after testosterone exposure report some differences as compared to ovaries without such exposure, although it is difficult to ascertain if these characteristics have functional impacts beyond their roles as likely biomarkers of increased ovarian testosterone exposure.

Limited studies report follicular reserve after testosterone as evaluated by anti-müllerian hormone (AMH) levels. In a prospective study of transgender patients starting testosterone, a significant decrease in AMH of 0.71 ng/mL from baseline (median 4.99 ng/mL) was noted after 12 months on testosterone. However, this

3 Effects of Masculinizing Therapy on Reproductive Capacity

Table 3.1 Comparison of histological ovarian changes with testosterone

Author, year	Polycystic ovary morphology (PCOM)?	Follicular phenotype	Tunica albuginea or outer cortex collagenization	Stromal hyperplasia	Stromal luteinization	CL or CA
Amirikia et al. [11]		Thickened basal membrane atretic follicles	✓			No recent
Futterweit and Deligdisch [12]	PCOM (13/19)	Multiple cystic follicles (17/19)	✓ (13/19)	✓ (16/19)	(5/19)	CL (3/19) CA (5/19)
Miller et al. [13]		Follicular cysts (32/32)				CL (4/32) CA (32/32)
Spinder et al. [14]	PCOM (18/26)	Multiple cystic follicles (18/26)	✓ (25/26)	✓ (21/26)	(7/26)	CL (4/26) CA (26/26)
Pache et al. [15]	PCOM	2x cystic follicles, 3.5x atretic follicles	✓ (16/17)	✓ (17/17)	✓ (12/17)	
Chadha et al. [16]		Increased cystic/atretic follicles	✓	✓	✓	
Grynberg et al. [17]	PCOM (89/112)	>12 antral follicles/ovary (89/112)		✓ (112/112)		
Ikeda et al. [18]	No PCOM	Similar preantral/antral follicles, more atretic transmen	✓ (10/11)	✓ (8/11)	✓ (10/11)	CL (0/11) CA (3/11)
Loverro et al. [19]		Multifollicular (10/12)				CL (2/10)
Khalifa et al. [20]		Bilateral cystic follicles (23/23)				CL (1/23)
Lin et al. [21]		Multiple bilateral cystic follicles (20/35)		(5/35)		CL (5/35)

decrease was accounted for by the 27 transgender patients with prior PCOS and not seen for the 27 without prior PCOS [10]. In two studies in which participants were on medications in addition to testosterone that may alter their AMH levels, one found no differences in AMH from baseline (with a progestin, [24]) while another found that AMH decreased (with an aromatase inhibitor and a gonadotropin-releasing hormone agonist, [25]). Promisingly, primordial follicles have been found in ovarian cortical histology for transgender men on testosterone and oocytes collected during oophorectomies have developed normal metaphase II spindles when matured in vitro [26, 27].

Most but not all individuals taking physiological doses of testosterone experience menstrual suppression. The observation of the occasional corpora lutea or corpora albicantia in ovaries during testosterone therapy suggests that some individuals may still occasionally ovulate [12–14, 18–21]. A 12-week study with 22 transmasculine individuals on testosterone utilized 3 days of elevated urinary pregnanediol-3-glucoronide as a proxy for ovulation. They found one individual with well-defined ovulation and 7 individuals with transient rises suggestive of dysfunctional ovulatory cycles. Most of these were observed in the month after testosterone initiation, but 2 transient rises were noted after 7+ and 13+ months of testosterone therapy [28]. This pattern of menstrual suppression with occasional breakthrough events is further supported by reports of pregnancies conceived while individuals were amenorrheic from testosterone [9] and highlights that testosterone alone is not considered sufficient contraception.

Data gathered from these observational studies has been limited by variations in testosterone administration regimens and serum levels achieved, as well as a wide range of testosterone exposure durations. Although rarely documented in the literature, it is also worth considering that some surgeons may have had their patients stop testosterone for a short period of time before surgeries and histopathological comparisons may not account for these pauses [16]. Further confounders include high rates of PCOS observed in transmasculine individuals prior to starting testosterone [29–31]. Questions remain regarding the reversibility and functional implications of testosterone-induced ovarian changes.

Impact of Testosterone on the Uterus

Conflicting uterine findings have been reported with testosterone. Differences between and within studies suggest that uterine findings between individuals may vary. One study of 112 individuals reported roughly half proliferative endometria (54/112) and half atrophic endometria (50/112) [17]. Another found a similar mix of active (proliferative 33/81, secretory 3/81) and atrophic/inactive (41/81) endometria [32]. Others found a majority of active endometria (proliferative in 61/94 and secretory in 4/94), although about a quarter had atrophic endometria (23/94) [33]. Similarly, another study reported active or secretory endometria in all 12 individuals studied [19]. In contrast, a study of 27 individuals found all inactive endometria [34], and a study of 40 individuals had a majority of inactive endometria (30/40) and a quarter with active endometria (7/40 proliferative, 3/40 secretory) [21]. Other notable uterine findings included cervical atrophy [13], endometrial stromal fibrosis and tubal metaplasia [21], and reduced proliferation marker expression [34]. Similar to ovarian studies, uterine comparisons are also limited by differences in testosterone regimen, durational variability, and possible brief hormonal pauses before surgery. Persistent bleeding on testosterone has been noted for a small fraction of individuals (12/52) as well as intermittent pelvic pain or cramping on testosterone (30/52) [33]. Encouragingly, studies where individuals have paused testosterone for reproductive purposes suggest that all or most individuals resumed menses with testosterone cessation, although the time course for this resumption has not been well characterized [6, 7, 9, 35, 36].

Impact of Testosterone on the Fallopian Tubes

Studies on fallopian tube changes with testosterone exposure are very limited. Androgen receptor expression has been observed in human tubal epithelium, suggesting testosterone can act directly on this tissue [37]. A study of 9 transgender men found that tubal ampulla had viscous luminal secretions and cellular debris with an increase in ciliated cells, in comparison to 19 cycling control patients with open ampullary lumen during the proliferative phase and watery secretions around ovulation turning more viscous during the secretory phase. Individuals treated with testosterone (7 out of 9) showed partial to complete closure of the lumen of the isthmus, while control patients had an isthmus that was generally clear and open [37]. The authors suggest that tubal flushing could potentially be a therapeutic measure following testosterone therapy for individuals aiming to conceive [37]. An earlier scanning electron microscope study of three individuals on testosterone noted a qualitative reduction in ciliated cells in the distal fimbriae and ampulla, with similar cilia in the isthmic and intramural tube regions [38]. Short-term in vitro exposure of human fallopian tube epithelium to testosterone resulted in reduced cilia beating and reduced transcript levels for key cilia regulators [39]. The reversibility of testosterone-induced changes in fallopian tubes has also not been investigated. Testosterone-induced fallopian tube changes will be more relevant to individuals pausing testosterone to try to conceive with minimal intervention and less relevant to those harvesting oocytes using assisted reproduction.

Pregnancies After Testosterone Therapy

Multiple pregnancies have been reported in the literature in which the transmasculine individual was the gestational parent or the oocyte donor after prolonged testosterone (Table 3.2). Typically, these are case reports or smaller studies and do not discuss individuals who were attempting pregnancy and may have been unsuccessful. Of note, testosterone is contraindicated in pregnancy [2] and it is recommended for testosterone to be paused prior to attempting conception. While studies to date are encouraging, additional data from larger studies are needed to investigate pregnancy outcomes after multiple durations of testosterone therapy and to study offspring resulting from testosterone-exposed oocytes.

Table 3.2 Pregnancies after prior testosterone (T) use

Author, Year	# of Pregnancies after T therapy	Additional notes
Ellis et al. [40]	6	Qualitative study, screened for a successful birth. Of 8 male-identified or gender-variant gestational parents, 6 had used T, and 4 had experienced at least 1 miscarriage.
Light et al. [9]	25	Survey of transgender men with successful birth. Of those who with prior T, 21/25 used their own oocytes.
Broughton and Omurtag [36]	1 (partner carried)	Case report, 1 transgender man with IVF post T, ongoing pregnancy (partner).
Light et al. [8]	11	Survey on family planning and contraception. Includes multiple pregnancies/individual and 5 abortions.
Adeleye et al. [6]	3 (2 partner carried)	Retrospective chart review, includes 7 transgender men post T, 1 spontaneous abortion in transgender man, 1 ongoing pregnancy (partner).
Hahn et al. [41]	1	Case report, only a few months of T pre-pregnancy.
Leung et al. [7]	11 (8 partner carried)	Retrospective cohort study, prior T use in 6/7 who chose IVF with transfer. Numbers include multiple pregnancies/individual, 1 pregnancy that did not lead to live birth, 1 twin pregnancy, 2 ongoing pregnancies, and 1 individual without prior T.
Stroumsa et al. [42]	1	Case report, 1 transgender man, presented to emergency room not aware of pregnancy and in labor leading to stillbirth.
Amir et al. [43]	1 (surrogate carried)	Retrospective cohort study, includes 6 transgender men with prior T, 1 ongoing pregnancy (surrogate).
de Sousa Resende et al. [44]	1 (partner carried)	Case report, 1 transgender man, ongoing pregnancy (partner).
Falck et al. [45]	8	Qualitative study, transmasculine individuals who had given birth.
Greenwald et al. [46]	1 (partner carried)	Case report, 1 transgender man, IVF on T, partner carried.
Moseson et al. [47]	15	Survey of pregnancy intentions and outcomes in transgender, non-binary, and gender-expansive people, 15 pregnancies in 12 individuals after starting T. Of these, 4 pregnancies occurred while on T (2 ended in miscarriage, 1 abortion, and 1 unknown).
Yaish et al. [10]	7 (1 surrogate carried)	Prospective and cross-sectional study of ovarian reserve with T. Includes 3 transgender men with prior T that carried 6 children (one carried 4), and 1 who used a surrogate.

Assisted Reproductive Technology Outcomes After Testosterone

Over the last few years, there has been a notable increase in publications discussing assisted reproductive technology (ART) outcomes for transgender men (Table 3.3). Similar ART outcomes have been demonstrated in transgender men with prior

3 Effects of Masculinizing Therapy on Reproductive Capacity

Table 3.3 Assisted reproductive outcomes after initiation of testosterone (T)

Author, Year	# Patients with prior T Therapy	T washout duration	Outcomes	Key takeaways
[36]	1	3 months	16 oocytes retrieved, 13 mature, 7 mature oocytes fertilized with ICSI. Two blastocysts transferred to partner, ongoing pregnancy. One additional blastocyst cryopreserved (others lower quality).	Highlights potential for IVF after prior T. Discusses somewhat arbitrary 3-month washout.
[6]	7	Approximately 6 months	Lower peak estradiol and lower number of oocytes retrieved in transgender men with T as compared to transgender men without T and cisgender controls. Differences go away when 2 outliers with low antral follicle count <5 were removed. No differences in oocyte maturity rates. 3 pregnancies after prior T (2 with partners carrying, one ongoing, one spontaneous abortion in transgender man).	Similar outcomes after prior T as compared to control groups (with 2 outliers removed).
[7]	16	1–12 months	No statistically significant differences between transgender patients with prior T and matched 130 cisgender controls (in age, AMH, oocytes retrieved, oocyte maturity, peak estradiol). 6 couples with prior T achieved live birth.	Similar outcomes after prior T as compared to control groups.
[43]	6	5–21 months	No differences in oocytes retrieved, MII oocytes, oocyte maturity rates, or peak estradiol between transgender men with prior T as compared to transgender men without prior T and fertile cisgender women. Embryo cryopreservation for 5 of 6 with prior T yielded good-quality embryos, and one ongoing surrogate pregnancy.	Similar outcomes after prior T as compared to control groups including fertile cisgender women.

(continued)

Table 3.3 (continued)

Author, Year	# Patients with prior T Therapy	T washout duration	Outcomes	Key takeaways
[48]	1	7 days	13 oocytes retrieved, 11 mature were vitrified.	Demonstrates feasibility of short duration of T cessation prior to oocyte cryopreservation.
[49]	1	3 months (for round 1)	Round 1: 11 oocytes retrieved, 10 cryopreserved (6 MII, 4 GV). Round 2: 14 oocytes retrieved, 13 cryopreserved (6 MII, 1 M1, 6 GV)	Highlights potential for oocyte cryopreservation after prior T therapy.
[44]	1	Possibly until return of menses	16 oocytes retrieved, 12 mature oocytes. ICSI (8 2PN, one 1PN, 3 non fertilized). One blastocyst transferred to partner, ongoing pregnancy. 5 embryos cryopreserved.	Highlights potential for IVF after prior T therapy.
[46]	1	No washout: Continuous T	20 oocytes retrieved, 16 mature, 13 fertilized with ICSI. 5 blastocysts, only one chromosomally normally, transferred to partner, leading to developmentally normal 2-year-old.	Report of live birth with continuous use of T. Indications for further study given high aneuploidy rate.
[50]	83	No washout: Ovarian tissue oocyte IVM on T	Mean of 23 ± 15.8 COCs per participant were collected. In vitro maturation rate 23.8%, vitrification rate 21.5%, survival after warming 72.6%. ICSI in 139 oocytes, 34.5% fertilization, 52.1% reached day 3. One blastocyst on day 5. Aberrant cleavage in 45.8% and early embryo arrest in 91.7%. Normal genetic pattern in 42%.	Low efficiency ovarian tissue oocyte IVM for patients on T.

testosterone exposure as compared to transgender men without prior testosterone use and cisgender women [6, 7, 43]. These 3 comparison studies in combination with multiple case reports [36, 44, 49] collectively support the use of ART after pausing testosterone. Recent case reports also demonstrate successful oocyte collection after a minimal testosterone washout period [48] as well as successful oocyte collection, fertilization, and live birth without pausing testosterone [46]. A paradigm that does not require testosterone cessation could remove a major hurdle to use of these assisted reproductive technologies. To support patient well-being,

3 Effects of Masculinizing Therapy on Reproductive Capacity

clinicians may also include aromatase inhibitors in parallel with gonadotropin stimulation to reduce elevations of estradiol and utilize transabdominal ultrasounds when possible [51]. Ovarian tissue cryopreservation at the time of a gender-affirming oophorectomy may also be a practical option for transgender men that would remove the need for ovarian stimulation. A recent study has also investigated the approach of ovarian tissue oocyte in vitro maturation (IVM) for patients on testosterone and found it to have low efficiency [50]. More comparative studies are needed, particularly addressing the use or avoidance of prolonged testosterone cessation prior to oocyte collection. A more extensive review of fertility and fertility preservation options for transmasculine people is presented in Chap. 4.

Animal Models for Gender-Affirming Testosterone

Animal models with a specific focus on masculinizing testosterone therapy are relatively new. In this section we describe findings from several recent mouse studies aimed at understanding the influence of masculinizing testosterone on reproduction. We also discuss relevant findings from PCOS animal model research and some of the limitations of the organizational/activational dichotomy.

The first mouse model aimed at understanding effects of gender-affirming testosterone used ovariectomized mice to study atherosclerosis and bone health and thus analyses of reproductive function could not be performed [52, 53]. To allow for reproductive analyses, we created a mouse model of masculinizing testosterone using mice with intact reproductive axes [54]. Adult female C57BL/6N mice treated with testosterone enanthate injections twice weekly for 6 weeks stopped having estrous cycles, showed clitoromegaly, no evidence of corpus lutea formation, and an increase in atretic cyst-like late antral follicles as compared to controls. Encouragingly, there were no detectable differences in the number of primordial, primary, secondary, or total antral follicles between control mice and those treated with testosterone for 6 weeks [54]. This suggests that testosterone may not have a major impact on ovarian reserve, and there may be a pool of unaffected early follicles from which to recruit. Recently, another group built on this work and used in vitro fertilization to compare CF-1 mice injected with testosterone cypionate once weekly for 6 weeks [55]. They noted similar acyclicity and clitoromegaly and found a reduction in corpora lutea with similar numbers of antral and atretic follicles between testosterone-treated mice and controls [55]. Encouragingly, they performed ovarian stimulation and found similar numbers of ovulated oocytes fertilizable to the two-cell stage in mice both on testosterone and after a period of testosterone cessation as compared to controls [55]. This supports the emerging practice of performing oocyte harvesting without having individuals pause their testosterone [51]. For those interested in pausing testosterone to carry a pregnancy, we have also characterized the reversibility of testosterone-induced acyclicity after 6 weeks of treatment with a testosterone enanthate pellet, demonstrating a prompt return of cyclic ovulatory function with corpora lutea formation after well-defined testosterone cessation [56]. Future animal model work will need to address longer durations of testosterone therapy and multiple fertility metrics.

Animal models have also been helpful in elucidating neuroendocrine mechanisms for androgen-induced cycle suppression. A 2020 study with ovariectomized young adult female mice treated for 2 weeks with implants of the non-aromatizable androgen, dihydrotestosterone (DHT) found reduced LH pulsatility in DHT-treated mice as compared to controls with decreased frequency, amplitude, peak, basal, and mean LH levels [57]. They also found suppression of *Kiss1* and *Tac2* gene expression in the arcuate nucleus of the hypothalamus for DHT-treated mice [57]. As gonadotropin-releasing hormone neurons do not express the androgen receptor, the negative feedback from androgens may be due to downregulation of these upstream positive regulators, kisspeptin and neurokinin-B. In addition to the hypothalamus, they also reported reduced LH secretion with gonadotropin-releasing hormone (GnRH) pulse treatment in DHT-treated in vitro pituitaries [57]. Ultimately, these results suggest that androgens can provide negative feedback to female gonadotropin release at both the hypothalamic and pituitary levels.

Historically, animal model research aimed at understanding the consequences of androgens on reproduction has focused on PCOS. For many PCOS animal models, hormone doses are lower than would typically be used for gender-affirming testosterone and hormones are administered in the prenatal or prepubertal periods. In contrast, the majority of transmasculine individuals taking testosterone are postpubertal. Long-term research understanding the influence of sex steroids, such as testosterone, on adults is fairly rare. Sex steroid changes have been historically understood by an organizational/activational paradigm. In this paradigm, organizational (permanent) changes can occur during development (prenatal, prepubertal periods) and only activational (transient) changes occur in adults. An over-reliance on the strict dichotomy of the organizational/activational framework has likely limited study of sex steroid changes on adults [58]. PCOS animal model studies have been extensively reviewed, with species including mice, rats, sheep, and monkeys and PCOS-inducing treatments including androgens (DHT, dehydroepiandrosterone, testosterone), estrogen, aromatase inhibitors, antiprogestins, constant light exposure, as well as transgenic models [59–63]. Researchers have also focused on the complex roles of androgens in normal and pathological ovarian function, particularly regarding lessons learned from androgen receptor knockout models [64, 65]. Of these studies, there are a few focused on PCOS that have used relevant postpubertal androgen administration.

In a relevant postpubertal model, reduced fertility and acyclicity were seen in DHT-treated mice as compared to controls, but reversibility following DHT cessation was not examined [66]. Another mouse study found reversibility 30 days post cessation of DHT-induced stromal changes and lack of corporal lutea, although DHT treatment began in the peripubertal period [67]. Notably, DHT differs from testosterone in that it is not aromatizable to estradiol and is not used clinically for masculinization. A recent study comparing 12 weeks of DHT and testosterone treatments in peripubertal mice found similar PCOS-like reproductive changes in both, but markedly more metabolic changes in DHT-treated wild-type mice as compared to those treated with testosterone [68]. Notably, when they then compared androgen receptor knockout mice, testosterone induced some reproductive changes while DHT did not, suggesting that both androgenic and estrogenic pathways likely mediate testosterone-induced reproductive alterations [68]. Despite key differences in PCOS and gender-affirming testosterone, there is meaningful research overlap due to methodological similarities in their respective animal models.

Unanswered Questions

Despite increasing research attention, multiple unanswered questions remain with regard to transmasculine reproduction. Studies present contrasting findings regarding the impact of testosterone on the reproductive tract, including the ovaries, uterus, and fallopian tubes. The functional impact of any testosterone-induced changes and their reversibility if testosterone is paused for reproductive purposes has not been well established. Although studies suggest the possibility of fertility for at least some after testosterone therapy, whether this is a something individuals can expect remains to be determined. Additionally, for those choosing ovarian stimulation with oocyte collection, questions remain regarding the option of remaining on testosterone during this process and/or the optimal duration for pausing testosterone prior to stimulation. As more answers emerge from ongoing research efforts, clinical guidelines will hopefully provide more nuance regarding reproductive options after prolonged testosterone exposure.

References

1. Hembree WC, Cohen-Kettenis PT, Gooren L, Hannema SE, Meyer WJ, Murad MH, Rosenthal SM, Safer JD, Tangpricha V, T'Sjoen GG. Endocrine treatment of gender-dysphoric/gender-incongruent persons: an Endocrine Society* clinical practice guideline. J Clin Endocrinol Metab. 2017;102:1–35.
2. Coleman E, Bockting W, Botzer M, Cohen-Kettenis P, DeCuypere G, Feldman J, Fraser L, Green J, Knudson G, Meyer WJ, et al. Standards of Care for the Health of transsexual, transgender, and gender-nonconforming people, version 7. Int J Transgenderism. 2011;13:165–232.
3. Ethics Committee of the American Society for Reproductive Medicine. Access to fertility services by transgender persons: an Ethics Committee opinion. Fertil Steril. 2015;104:1111–5. Elsevier.
4. Auer MK, Fuss J, Nieder TO, Briken P, Biedermann SV, Stalla GK, Beckmann MW, Hildebrandt T. Desire to have children among transgender people in Germany: a cross-sectional multi-center study. J Sex Med. 2018;15:757–67.
5. Baram S, Myers SA, Yee S, Librach CL. Fertility preservation for transgender adolescents and young adults: a systematic review. Hum Reprod Update. 2019;25:694–716.
6. Adeleye AJ, Cedars MI, Smith J, Mok-Lin E. Ovarian stimulation for fertility preservation or family building in a cohort of transgender men. J Assist Reprod Genet. 2019;36:2155–61.
7. Leung A, Sakkas D, Pang S, Thornton K, Resetkova N. Assisted reproductive technology outcomes in female-to-male transgender patients compared with cisgender patients: a new frontier in reproductive medicine. Fertil Steril. 2019;112:858–65.

8. Light A, Wang LF, Zeymo A, Gomez-Lobo V. Family planning and contraception use in transgender men. Contraception. 2018;98:266–9.
9. Light AD, Obedin-Maliver J, Sevelius JM, Kerns JL. Transgender men who experienced pregnancy after female-to-male gender transitioning. Obstet Gynecol. 2014;124:1120–7.
10. Yaish I, Tordjman K, Amir H, Malinger G, Salemnick Y, Shefer G, Serebro M, Azem F, Golani N, Sofer Y, et al. Functional ovarian reserve in transgender men receiving testosterone therapy: evidence for preserved anti-Müllerian hormone and antral follicle count under prolonged treatment. Hum Reprod. 2021;36:2753–60.
11. Amirikia H, Savoy-Moore RT, Sundareson AS, Moghissi KS. The effects of long-term androgen treatment on the ovary. Fertil Steril. 1986;45:202–8.
12. Futterweit W, Deligdisch L. Histopathological effects of exogenously administered testosterone in 19 female to male transsexuals. J Clin Endocrinol Metab. 1986;62:16–21.
13. Miller N, Bédard YC, Cooter NB, Shaul DL. Histological changes in the genital tract in transsexual women following androgen therapy. Histopathology. 1986;10:661–9.
14. Spinder T, Spijkstra JJ, van den Tweel JG, Burger CW, van Kessel H, Hompes PGA, Gooren LJG. The effects of long term testosterone administration on pulsatile luteinizing hormone secretion and on ovarian histology in Eugonadal female to male transsexual subjects. J Clin Endocrinol Metab. 1989;69:151–7.
15. Pache TD, Chadha S, Gooren LJG, Hop WCJ, Jaarsma KW, Dommerholt HBR, Fauser BCJM. Ovarian morphology in long-term androgen-treated female to male transsexuals. A human model for the study of polycystic ovarian syndrome? Histopathology. 1991;19:445–52.
16. Chadha S, Pache TD, Huikeshoven FJM, Brinkmann AO, van der Kwast TH. Androgen receptor expression in human ovarian and uterine tissue of long term androgen-treated transsexual women. Hum Pathol. 1994;25:1198–204.
17. Grynberg M, Fanchin R, Dubost G, Colau JC, Brémont-Weil C, Frydman R, Ayoubi J-M. Histology of genital tract and breast tissue after long-term testosterone administration in a female-to-male transsexual population. Reprod Biomed Online. 2010;20:553–8.
18. Ikeda K, Baba T, Noguchi H, Nagasawa K, Endo T, Kiya T, Saito T. Excessive androgen exposure in female-to-male transsexual persons of reproductive age induces hyperplasia of the ovarian cortex and stroma but not polycystic ovary morphology. Hum Reprod. 2013;28:453–61.
19. Loverro G, Resta L, Dellino M, Edoardo DN, Cascarano MA, Loverro M, Mastrolia SA. Uterine and ovarian changes during testosterone administration in young female-to-male transsexuals. Taiwan J Obstet Gynecol. 2016;55:686–91.
20. Khalifa MA, Toyama A, Klein ME, Santiago V. Histologic features of hysterectomy specimens from female-male transgender individuals. Int J Gynecol Pathol. 2019;38:520–7.
21. Lin LH, Hernandez A, Marcus A, Deng F-M, Adler E. Histologic findings in gynecologic tissue from Transmasculine individuals undergoing gender-affirming surgery. Arch Patholol Lab Med. 2021;146:742.
22. Hughesdon PE. Morphology and Morphogenesis of the Stein-Leventhal Ovary and of So-called "Hyperthecosis". Obstet Gynecol Surv. 1982;37:59–77.
23. Caanen MR, Schouten NE, Kuijper EAM, van Rijswijk J, van den Berg MH, van Dulmen-den Broeder E, Overbeek A, van Leeuwen FE, van Trotsenburg M, Lambalk CB. Effects of long-term exogenous testosterone administration on ovarian morphology, determined by transvaginal (3D) ultrasound in female-to-male transsexuals. Hum Reprod. 2017;32:1457–64.
24. Tack LJW, Craen M, Dhondt K, Vanden BH, Laridaen J, Cools M. Consecutive lynestrenol and cross-sex hormone treatment in biological female adolescents with gender dysphoria: a retrospective analysis. Biol Sex Differ. 2016;7:14.
25. Caanen MR, Soleman RS, Kuijper EAM, Kreukels BPC, De Roo C, Tilleman K, De Sutter P, van Trotsenburg MAA, Broekmans FJ, Lambalk CB. Antimüllerian hormone levels decrease in female-to-male transsexuals using testosterone as cross-sex therapy. Fertil Steril. 2015;103:1340–5.
26. Lierman S, Tilleman K, Braeckmans K, Peynshaert K, Weyers S, T'Sjoen G, De Sutter P. Fertility preservation for trans men: frozen-thawed in vitro matured oocytes collected at

the time of ovarian tissue processing exhibit normal meiotic spindles. J Assist Reprod Genet. 2017;34:1449–56.

27. De Roo C, Lierman S, Tilleman K, Peynshaert K, Braeckmans K, Caanen M, Lambalk CB, Weyers S, T'Sjoen G, Cornelissen R, et al. Ovarian tissue cryopreservation in female-to-male transgender people: insights into ovarian histology and physiology after prolonged androgen treatment. Reprod Biomed Online. 2017;34:557–66.

28. Taub RL, Ellis SA, Neal-Perry G, Magaret AS, Prager SW, Micks EA. The effect of testosterone on ovulatory function in transmasculine individuals. Am J Obstet Gynecol. 2020;223:229.e1–8.

29. Baba T, Endo T, Honnma H, Kitajima Y, Hayashi T, Ikeda H, Masumori N, Kamiya H, Moriwaka O, Saito T. Association between polycystic ovary syndrome and female-to-male transsexuality. Hum Reprod. 2007;22:1011–6.

30. Becerra-Fernández A, Pérez-López G, Román MM, Martín-Lazaro JF, Pérez MJL, Araque NA, Rodríguez-Molina JM, Sertucha MCB, Vilas MVA. Prevalence of hyperandrogenism and polycystic ovary syndrome in female to male transsexuals. Endocrinol Nutr. 2014;61:351–8.

31. Mueller A, Gooren LJ, Naton-Schötz S, Cupisti S, Beckmann MW, Dittrich R. Prevalence of polycystic ovary syndrome and Hyperandrogenemia in female-to-male transsexuals. J Clin Endocrinol Metab. 2008;93:1408–11.

32. Hawkins M, Deutsch MB, Obedin-Maliver J, Stark B, Grubman J, Jacoby A, Jacoby VL. Endometrial findings among transgender and gender nonbinary people using testosterone at the time of gender-affirming hysterectomy. Fertil Steril. 2021;115:1312–7.

33. Grimstad FW, Fowler KG, New EP, Ferrando CA, Pollard RR, Chapman G, Gomez-Lobo V, Gray M. Uterine pathology in transmasculine persons on testosterone: a retrospective multi-center case series. Am J Obstet Gynecol. 2019;220:257.e1–7.

34. Perrone AM, Cerpolini S, Maria Salfi NC, Ceccarelli C, De GLB, Formelli G, Casadio P, Ghi T, Pelusi G, Pelusi C, et al. Effect of long-term testosterone administration on the endometrium of female-to-male (FtM) transsexuals. J Sex Med. 2009;6:3193–200.

35. Armuand G, Dhejne C, Olofsson JII, Rodriguez-Wallberg KAA. Transgender men's experiences of fertility preservation: a qualitative study. Hum Reprod. 2017;32:383–90.

36. Broughton D, Omurtag K. Care of the transgender or gender-nonconforming patient undergoing in vitro fertilization. Int J Transgenderism. 2017;18:372–5.

37. Dulohery K, Trottmann M, Bour S, Liedl B, Alba-Alejandre I, Reese S, Hughes B, Stief CG, Kölle S. How do elevated levels of testosterone affect the function of the human fallopian tube and fertility?—New insights. Mol Reprod Dev. 2020;87:30–44.

38. Patek E, Nilsson L, Johannisson E, Hellema M, Bout J. Scanning electron microscopic study of the human fallopian tube. Report III. The effect of Midpregnancy and of various steroids. Fertil Steril. 1973;24:31–43.

39. Jackson-Bey T, Colina J, Isenberg BC, Coppeta J, Urbanek M, Kim JJ, Woodruff TK, Burdette JE, Russo A. Exposure of human fallopian tube epithelium to elevated testosterone results in alteration of cilia gene expression and beating. Hum Reprod. 2020;35:2086–96.

40. Ellis SA, Wojnar DM, Pettinato M. Conception, pregnancy, and birth experiences of male and gender variant gestational parents: It's how we could have a family. J Midwifery Women's Heal. 2015;60:62–9.

41. Hahn M, Sheran N, Weber S, Cohan D, Obedin-Maliver J. Providing patient-centered perinatal Care for Transgender men and Gender-Diverse Individuals. Obstet Gynecol. 2019;134:959–63.

42. Stroumsa D, Roberts EF, Kinnear H, Harris LH. The power and limits of classification – a 32-year-old man with abdominal pain. N Engl J Med. 2019;380:1885–8.

43. Amir H, Yaish I, Samara N, Hasson J, Groutz A, Azem F. Ovarian stimulation outcomes among transgender men compared with fertile cisgender women. J Assist Reprod Genet. 2020;37:2463–72.

44. de Sousa Resende S, Kussumoto VH, Arima FHC, Krul PC, Rodovalho NCM, Jesus Sampaio MR, de Alves MM. A transgender man, a cisgender woman, and assisted reproductive technologies: a Brazilian case report. J Bras Reprod Assist. 2020;24:513–6.

45. Falck F, Frisén L, Dhejne C, Armuand G. Undergoing pregnancy and childbirth as trans masculine in Sweden: experiencing and dealing with structural discrimination, gender norms and microaggressions in antenatal care, delivery and gender clinics. Int J Transgender Heal. 2020;22:42–53.
46. Greenwald P, Dubois B, Lekovich J, Pang JH, Safer J. Successful in vitro fertilization in a cisgender female carrier using oocytes retrieved from a transgender man maintained on testosterone. AACE Clin Case Reports. 2021;8:7–9.
47. Moseson H, Fix L, Hastings J, Stoeffler A, Lunn MR, Flentje A, Lubensky ME, Capriotti MR, Ragosta S, Forsberg H, et al. Pregnancy intentions and outcomes among transgender, nonbinary, and gender-expansive people assigned female or intersex at birth in the United States: results from a national, quantitative survey. Int J Transgender Heal. 2021;22:30–41.
48. Cho K, Harjee R, Roberts J, Dunne C. Fertility preservation in a transgender man without prolonged discontinuation of testosterone: a case report and literature review. F&S Rep. 2020;1:43–7.
49. Insogna IG, Ginsburg E, Srouji S. Fertility preservation for adolescent transgender male patients: a case series. J Adolesc Health. 2020;66:750–3.
50. Lierman S, Tolpe A, De Croo I, De Gheselle S, Defreyne J, Baetens M, Dheedene A, Colman R, Menten B, T'Sjoen G, et al. Low feasibility of in vitro matured oocytes originating from cumulus complexes found during ovarian tissue preparation at the moment of gender confirmation surgery and during testosterone treatment for fertility preservation in transgender men. Fertil Steril. 2021;116:1068–76.
51. Moravek MB, Kinnear HM, George J, Batchelor J, Shikanov A, Padmanabhan V, Randolph JF. Impact of exogenous testosterone on reproduction in transgender men. Endocrinology. 2020;161:1–13.
52. Goetz LG, Mamillapalli R, Devlin MJ, Robbins AE, Majidi-Zolbin M, Taylor HS. Cross-sex testosterone therapy in ovariectomized mice: addition of low-dose estrogen preserves bone architecture. Am J Physiol - Endocrinol Metab. 2017;313:E540–51.
53. Goetz LG, Mamillapalli R, Sahin C, Majidi-Zolbin M, Ge G, Mani A, Taylor HS. Addition of estradiol to cross-sex testosterone therapy reduces atherosclerosis plaque formation in female ApoE−/− mice. Endocrinology. 2018;159:754–62.
54. Kinnear HM, Constance ES, David A, Marsh EE, Padmanabhan V, Shikanov A, Moravek MB. A mouse model to investigate the impact of testosterone therapy on reproduction in transgender men. Hum Reprod. 2019;34:2009–17.
55. Bartels CB, Uliasz TF, Lestz L, Mehlmann LM. Short-term testosterone use in female mice does not impair fertilizability of eggs: implications for the fertility care of transgender males. Hum Reprod. 2020;36:1–10.
56. Kinnear HM, Hashim PH, Dela CC, Rubenstein G, Chang FL, Nimmagadda L, Brunette MA, Padmanabhan V, Shikanov A, Moravek MB. Reversibility of testosterone-induced acyclicity after testosterone cessation in a transgender mouse model. F&S Sci. 2021;2:116–23.
57. Esparza LA, Terasaka T, Lawson MA, Kauffman AS. Androgen suppresses in vivo and in vitro LH pulse secretion and neural Kiss1 and Tac2 gene expression in female mice. Endocrinology. 2020;161:1–16.
58. Arnold AP, Breedlove SM. Organizational and Activational effects of sex steroids on brain and behavior: a reanalysis. Horm Behav. 1985;19:469–98.
59. Abbott DH, Barnett DK, Bruns CM, Dumesic DA. Androgen excess fetal programming of female reproduction: a developmental aetiology for polycystic ovary syndrome? Hum Reprod Update. 2005;11:357–74.
60. van Houten ELAF, Visser JA. Mouse models to study polycystic ovary syndrome: a possible link between metabolism and ovarian function? Reprod Biol. 2014;14:32–43.
61. Padmanabhan V, Veiga-Lopez A. Animal models of the polycystic ovary syndrome phenotype. Steroids. 2013;78:734–40.

62. Shi D, Vine DF. Animal models of polycystic ovary syndrome: a focused review of rodent models in relationship to clinical phenotypes and cardiometabolic risk. Fertil Steril. 2012;98:185–93.
63. Walters KA, Allan CM, Handelsman DJ. Rodent models for human polycystic ovary syndrome. Biol Reprod. 2012;86:1–12.
64. Walters KA. Role of androgens in normal and pathological ovarian function. Reproduction. 2015;149:R193–218.
65. Walters KA, Paris VR, Aflatounian A, Handelsman DJ. Androgens and ovarian function: translation from basic discovery research to clinical impact. J Endocrinol. 2019;242:R23–50.
66. Ma Y, Andrisse S, Chen Y, Childress S, Xue P, Wang Z, Jones D, Ko C, Divall S, Wu S. Androgen receptor in the ovary theca cells plays a critical role in androgen-induced reproductive dysfunction. Endocrinology. 2017;158:98–108.
67. Sun L-F, Yang Y-L, Xiao T-X, Li M-X, Zhang JV. Removal of DHT can relieve polycystic ovarian but not metabolic abnormalities in DHT-induced hyperandrogenism in mice. Reprod Fertil Dev. 2019;31:1597–606.
68. Aflatounian A, Edwards MC, Rodriguez Paris V, Bertoldo MJ, Desai R, Gilchrist RB, Ledger WL, Handelsman DJ, Walters KA. Androgen signaling pathways driving reproductive and metabolic phenotypes in a PCOS mouse model. J Endocrinol. 2020;245:381–95.

Chapter 4
Fertility and Fertility Preservation in Transmasculine Individuals

Brett Stark, Viji Sundaram, and Evelyn Mok-Lin

Introduction

TGNB people desire to have children for the same reasons as others including intimacy, nurturance, and family [1]; however, for these individuals, it may signify a deeper alignment of their gender expression through parenthood and achieving a desired sense of self [2]. While the right to procreate has traditionally been granted to fertile, heterosexual couples, the advent of assisted reproductive technologies (ART) has revolutionized reproductive options for infertile couples, LGBTQ couples, and single individuals desiring biologic parenthood [2].

Fertility preservation (FP) is the practice of taking definitive steps to improve the chances of biological reproduction in those who are predicted to have significant infertility [3]. The World Professional Association for Transgender Health (WPATH), Endocrine Society, and American Society of Reproduction (ASRM) all recommend counseling TGNB individuals on fertility options prior to any medical or surgical treatments [4], though there are few data implicating the adverse impact of gender-affirming treatment (GAT) on fertility outcomes [5].

Multiple factors should be considered when counseling transmasculine individuals on fertility and FP options, including age at referral, presence of dysphoria, anticipated timeline for gender-affirming therapy that might affect fertility, family-planning goals, partner's reproductive organs if partnered, and the individual (or partner's) desire to carry a pregnancy [6]. Additionally, it is important to counsel patients on the interventions required in order to use their cryopreserved gametes in the future and expected costs associated with these procedures [7].

B. Stark · E. Mok-Lin (✉)
University of California, San Francisco, CA, USA
e-mail: brett.stark@ucsf.edu; evelyn.mok-lin@ucsf.edu

V. Sundaram
Kaiser Permanente, San Francisco, CA, USA

© The Author(s), under exclusive license to Springer Nature
Switzerland AG 2023
M. B. Moravek, G. de Haan (eds.), *Reproduction in Transgender and Nonbinary Individuals*, https://doi.org/10.1007/978-3-031-14933-7_4

The objectives of this chapter are to discuss fertility and fertility preservation options available to adult and adolescent transmasculine persons.

Gender-Affirming Treatment and Fertility

A common course of medical therapy for gender dysphoric transmasculine individuals seeking intervention involves, depending on their age, the arrest of puberty with GnRH analogues at Tanner stage 2, addition of parenteral or transdermal T at approximately 16 years, and maintenance of physiologic levels in adulthood [8]. While surgical resection of the uterus and/or ovaries has clear and permanent deleterious effects on future reproduction, the effect of long-term testosterone on fertility is less evident [7, 9].

Animal models investigating ovarian histology following androgen exposure have mainly been studied in the context of polycystic ovary syndrome (PCOS) [10, 11]. Primate, sheep, and murine PCOS models have documented changes in ovarian histopathology and function; however, most of these studies have involved prenatal and prepubertal androgen exposure [5, 10]. A recent publication evaluated ovarian follicular morphology and corpora lutea counts with varying doses of subcutaneous testosterone injections in 20 female mice [12]. Testosterone-treated mice were found to have no reduction in primordial, primary, secondary, or total antral follicle counts compared to control mice, suggesting that testosterone therapy does not deplete the existing ovarian reserve [12]. Testosterone-treated animals also had an increase in atretic cyst-like late antral follicles, consistent with a PCO-morphology, and an absence of corpora lutea with lack of normal ovulatory cycles [12].

Human studies evaluating ovarian histological changes following testosterone exposure in individuals assigned female at birth have reported an ovarian phenotype similar to PCOS: increased collagenization of the tunica albuginea, stromal hyperplasia, and luteinization of stromal cells [13–15]. While some studies report polycystic follicles and antral follicle counts of more than 12 follicles per ovary, others report similar antral follicle counts between testosterone-treated transmasculine people and controls [13, 16]. Reported limitations of these studies include their observational nature, the variable length of time on testosterone prior to ovarian histological analysis, and the higher prevalence of PCOS (15–58%) at baseline in transmasculine people [7, 12]. The existing human studies of testosterone-treated individuals do not describe a direct effect on fertility or if testosterone-elicited changes are reversible upon cessation of therapy [7, 12].

For transmasculine patients initiating testosterone, amenorrhea typically occurs within 6 months [17, 18]. The timeline for resumption of menses upon discontinuation of testosterone is less clear, where some have suggested that it may even be irreversible for some [19]. In a cross-sectional study of 41 transgender men who became pregnant and delivered after transition, 25 (61%) reported testosterone use prior to pregnancy [20]. Those who chose to discontinue testosterone in preparation for a spontaneous pregnancy ($N = 20$) reported resumption of menses within

6 months, more commonly (*N* = 19) within 3 months [20]. Five transmasculine people became unintentionally pregnant while amenorrheic on testosterone [20]. While detailed length of time on testosterone was not described for these five individuals, data from this study as a whole irrefutably argue that transmasculine people on testosterone can retain fertility and become pregnant [20, 21]. Hence for transmasculine patients engaging in penetrative vaginal intercourse with a partner who produces sperm, contraception is recommended to prevent undesired pregnancies [22].

A more thorough review of what is known about the effects of gender-affirming testosterone on reproductive function is presented in Chap. 3.

Fertility Preservation in the Post-pubertal Transmasculine Individual

Initial steps should include a discussion regarding family-planning goals and timeline, reproductive function of partner if applicable, and patient and/or partner's desire to carry a pregnancy. Depending on these considerations, the mode and urgency of fertility preservation options can be determined. For individuals who have at least one ovary in situ, anti-müllerian hormone (AMH) and/or antral follicle count (AFC) may be used to assess ovarian reserve. AMH is beneficial as it does not vary with the menstrual cycle, and is a serum test that does not require special equipment or an experienced sonographer [23]. AFC, which closely correlates with AMH, is determined by counting the number of 2 to 10 mm follicles by transvaginal ultrasound [24]. While transmasculine individuals may be willing and able to undergo transvaginal ultrasound, transabdominal or transrectal ultrasounds should be considered depending on patient comfort and anatomy [3, 5, 25]. While transabdominal ultrasounds have been commonly cited as alternatives in the existing literature, few papers recommend the use of transrectal ultrasounds, which are overall well-tolerated, have adequate visualization of ovarian follicles comparable to transvaginal ultrasound, and are superior to transabdominal ultrasound [26, 27].

Traditionally, embryo cryopreservation has been used in cisgender females anticipating gonadotoxic radiation or chemotherapy [28]. While this may be feasible for some transmasculine people if they have a partner with sperm, this can be a major disadvantage to transmasculine people without access to a sperm source to fertilize oocytes at retrieval [28]. With improved vitrification techniques, oocyte cryopreservation has become a non-experimental option since 2012 and is routinely employed worldwide with equivalent pregnancy rates to fresh oocytes [29]. Oocyte cryopreservation following controlled ovarian stimulation (COS) is an excellent option for FP in postpubertal transmasculine people who anticipate gender-affirming interventions that will affect fertility such as testosterone or oophorectomy in the near future, or who do not plan to carry their own pregnancy [3].

Since 2014, multiple case reports describing oocyte cryopreservation in transmasculine individuals desiring FP have been published [30–32]. One observational study demonstrated that testosterone-naïve, post-pubertal transmasculine adolescents between the ages of 14 to 18 years had an average of 18.2 oocytes retrieved (range of 11–28y) [32]. Live births following oocyte vitrification pre-gender-affirming fertility-affecting intervention have been reported in the literature as well, including in two trans men who thawed their cryopreserved oocytes, fertilized with donor sperm, and transferred embryos into their cisgender female partners [31]. One couple had a monozygotic-diamniotic twin live birth after transfer of a euploid blast, and another had a dichorionic-diamniotic twin ongoing pregnancy following transfer of 2 day-5 embryos.

For transmasculine patients presenting for FP after initiation of testosterone, there are few publications to guide appropriate patient counseling regarding COS success following androgen use [12]. There are no professional guidelines specifying the duration or necessity of testosterone cessation prior to FP at this time. In the absence of data, the current practice for most clinicians is to temporarily suspend T treatment for an arbitrary length of time, usually between 1 to 6 months, or until resumption of menses [9, 20, 33]. Two recent studies report outcomes of patients with a history of testosterone use compared to cisgender women. Adeleye et al. reported on outcomes in a cohort of 13 transmasculine patients, 7 with a history of testosterone use for a median of 46 months [25]. Median discontinuation time for testosterone prior to COS was 6 months (range 1–13 months). Transmasculine patients with prior testosterone use had significantly fewer oocytes retrieved (median 12) than those never having used testosterone (median 25.5, $p = 0.038$), which lost significance when 2 outliers with diminished ovarian reserve (AFC < 5) were removed from the analysis. When comparing all transmasculine individuals to body-mass-index (BMI) matched cisgender women undergoing COS for either male factor infertility or elective FP, peak estradiol levels were noted to be statistically lower in transmasculine participants with no differences in total oocytes retrieved, number of mature oocytes, and all other cycle characteristics. In this study, three transmasculine individuals with prior testosterone use presented for additional family planning. Two desired transfer of embryos following donor insemination to their cisgender female partners, and 1 desired autologous transfer of embryos inseminated with their cisgender male partner's sperm. All 3 couples in the study became successfully pregnant.

Shortly thereafter, Leung et al. reported on ART outcomes in 26 transmasculine patients, 61% of whom had been on testosterone from 3 months to 17 years, compared to 130 age-, BMI-, and AMH-matched cisgender females [34]. All patients on testosterone were instructed to discontinue the medication and await menses. If a strong aversion to menses resumption was present, testosterone was discontinued with decreasing levels monitored until reaching the upper normal level of a cisgender female range. Participants stopped testosterone for a mean of 4 months (range 1–12 months) before COS start. Outcomes between cisgender and transmasculine participants interestingly showed statistically higher number of oocytes retrieved in the transmasculine group (19.9 ± 8.7) compared to the cisgender group

(15.9 ± 9.6), though higher total doses of gonadotropins were also used in the transmasculine group. Sub-analyses were performed between transmasculine individuals with prior testosterone use and cisgender females, which demonstrated that the number of oocytes retrieved trended higher in the transmasculine cohort, although the trend was not statistically significant. Investigators postulated that the higher number of oocytes in the transmasculine group may be due to the previously described PCOS-like biochemical environment with androgen use, leading to a high ovarian reserve and subsequent robust response to stimulation. This increased oocyte yield can also be seen in cisgender women with low ovarian reserve that are pretreated with testosterone before ART. It is thought that low doses of testosterone may improve follicular response and sensitivity to follicle-stimulating hormone [35]. Seven couples desiring pregnancy were described in the study. All seven ultimately became pregnant with deliveries of healthy children. While small and retrospective in nature, both of these studies suggest that follicular development and oocyte quality do not seem to be significantly impacted by prior testosterone use [25, 34].

While COS may be a viable option for many transmasculine individuals, it is not without major limitations. COS involves significant estrogen exposure with associated physical symptoms, frequent monitoring with pelvic ultrasound, and transvaginal aspiration of oocytes under sedation [36]. While these procedures alone can be traumatic to some transmasculine individuals, the physical changes associated with discontinuation of testosterone and elevated estradiol levels can be significantly dysphoric and a possible barrier to those seeking FP [33, 37]. Hence, there have been anecdotal reports, within our own institution as well as others, of transmasculine patients choosing to continue testosterone at the time of COS. One recently published case report demonstrated successful COS in a 28-year-old transmasculine individual with only 24 days of testosterone cessation [38]. He had been on testosterone for a total of 3 years, and ultimately had 11 mature oocytes retrieved. Earlier this year, a 20-year-old who had been on low-dose testosterone (25 mg IM weekly) for 18 months elected to continue throughout COS and had 22 mature oocytes retrieved [39]. This early data provide reassurance that COS and oocyte cryopreservation is possible without cessation of testosterone, although long-term quality and pregnancy outcomes are not yet available.

Additional methods for mitigation of dysphoric symptoms during this process include the use of transrectal or transabdominal ultrasounds as discussed above, and addition of aromatase inhibitors concurrently with gonadotropins to minimize estradiol elevations during COS, as described in breast cancer patients with estrogen-sensitive tumors [33, 40]. Sensitivity training for all healthcare professionals and office staff involved with regard to use of correct pronouns and preferred gender-specific terminology are also essential, as patients may report irritation and distress when others perceive them as women and use words such as "vagina," "ovaries," or "uterus" [33]. Notably, many of our patients have expressed no dysphoria with this process and do not require the offered mitigation techniques. A summary of options for fertility preservation in postpubertal transmasculine individuals can be found on Table 4.1.

Table 4.1 Options for fertility treatment in transmasculine individuals

	Fertility preservation	Fertility treatment
Postpubertal	1. Embryo cryopreservation with partner or donor sperm. 2. Oocyte cryopreservation.	1. IVF with partner/donor sperm and embryo transfer to self, partner, or gestational carrier.
Prepubertal	1. Ovarian tissue cryopreservation with autotransplantation. 2. Oocyte cryopreservation [experimental]. 3. Ovarian tissue cryopreservation with in vitro growth [future direction].	

Fertility Preservation in the Pre-pubertal Transmasculine Individual

With the recommendation to consider FP prior to the start of gender-affirming hormonal treatment, and increasing access to multidisciplinary models of care for TGNB people, there is a growing number of adolescents on pubertal suppressive agents presenting for discussion of FP prior to menarche [32, 41]. Pubertal suppression with a GnRH agonist has been well-documented as reversible, allowing reactivation of pubertal development and secondary sexual characteristics consistent with endogenous hormone production upon cessation of treatment [17, 42, 43]. However, most transmasculine patients will progress directly from puberty blockers to T, which poses a dilemma for FP in the setting of immature gametes. Until recently, pre-menarchal transmasculine individuals were counseled to consider ovarian tissue cryopreservation (OTC) as their only viable FP option, given that COS with oocyte retrieval was not known to be a possibility. In 2019, the first case of successful oocyte cryopreservation in a pre-menarchal patient was reported [44]. Four mature oocytes were retrieved after 30 days of gonadotropin injections from a 16-year-old transmasculine patient who had been on GnRH agonist since age 14. Subsequently, Insogna et al. reported a 15-year-old who had been on agonist since age 12, from whom 10 mature oocytes were retrieved after 11 days of medications [45]. While this novel technique is remarkable as a proof-of-concept and valuable as an additional FP option, data on oocyte quality and long-term outcomes do not exist and likely will not be available for many years given the young age of these individuals. Additionally, 2 to 4 weeks of gonadotropin injections, while shorter than initially hypothesized in the setting of ovarian suppression with GnRH agonist, may not be a viable physical, emotional, or financial option for some transmasculine adolescents and their families.

Considered experimental until 2019, OTC was typically reserved for pre-pubertal oncologic patients prior to gonadotoxic treatment or gonadectomy. Through this process, ovarian cortical tissue is removed laparoscopically without the need for gonadotropin injections, and cryopreserved for later orthotopic or heterotopic reimplantation into the same individual desiring a spontaneous pregnancy or IVF [46]. Over 130 live births have been reported worldwide from this technique; however, autotransplantation may not be an acceptable option for some TGNI individuals depending on their plans and feelings regarding their ovaries [46].

There has been increased recent interest in OTC in conjunction with in vitro maturation (IVM) as a feasible, though still experimental, option for adult transmasculine people electing for bilateral oophorectomy [7, 47]. Cumulus-oocyte complexes can be retrieved from frozen cortical ovarian tissue and subsequently matured in vitro with the creation of good quality embryos and reported live births [48, 49]. In trans masculine people who have been on testosterone for over a year, cortical follicle distribution is surprisingly normal and can be successfully in vitro matured [47, 50]. If routinely employed in transmasculine patients in the future, patients would not require an additional step for ovarian stimulation. For some this may prevent a situation in which they experience worsening dysphoria from the temporary change to an estrogen dominant hormonal milieu, but could rather be undertaken simultaneously at the time of gender-affirming oophorectomy [47, 50]. Much work is necessary before presenting this as a viable, routine option for transmasculine patients, particularly for prepubescent individuals for whom in vitro growth from primordial follicles would be required and has only been achieved in mice thus far [51]. A summary of options for fertility preservation in prepubertal transmasculine individuals can be found on Table 4.1.

The ethical implications of parents consenting for the reproductive rights of their children have been extensively discussed in oncologic cohorts, and must be addressed with this unique population of TGNB patients [52]. Youth have been described as overly influenced by short-term consequences, such as delayed hormonal therapy, as opposed to long-term issues such as fertility [53]. Hence, strategies to facilitate the informed consent process have been described that take into consideration an adolescent's maturity and decisional capacity [54]. Indeed, we have seen examples of young adolescent patients presenting for FP discussion with their parents, who are more concerned for preservation of fertility options for their child than the TGNB patient themselves. This raises concerns for parental consenting rights for invasive fertility procedures and autonomy of the child, which need to be explored in much more detail than currently exists in the literature [53, 54].

Conclusion

Research on the effects of long-term testosterone exposure on fertility and pregnancy outcomes are becoming increasingly available. While limited, data in animal models and clinical studies are reassuring thus far, with successful ovarian stimulation and live births in transmasculine individuals who have initiated testosterone. With increased awareness, legislative advocacy, and access to care, a growing number of transmasculine individuals are seeking fertility preservation counseling and treatment, and at younger ages. The majority of existing literature used to guide standards in TGNB fertility care are derived from retrospective analyses at single institutions. Significant, multi-institutional research studies are needed in order to provide informed, evidence-based counseling of TGNB individuals desiring genetic parenthood.

References

1. Access to fertility services by transgender persons. An ethics committee opinion. Fertil Steril. 2015;104(5):1111–5.
2. Condat A, Mendes N, Drouineaud V, Gründler N, Lagrange C, Chiland C, et al. Biotechnologies that empower transgender persons to self-actualize as individuals, partners, spouses, and parents are defining new ways to conceive a child: psychological considerations and ethical issues. Philos Ethics Humanit Med. 2018;13(1):1.
3. Mattawanon N, Spencer JB, Schirmer DA, Tangpricha V. Fertility preservation options in transgender people: a review. Rev Endocr Metab Disord. 2018;19(3):231–42.
4. Coleman E, Bockting W, Botzer M, Cohen-Kettenis P, DeCuypere G, Feldman J, et al. Standards of Care for the Health of transsexual, transgender, and gender-nonconforming people, version 7. Int J Transgenderism. 2012;13(4):165–232.
5. Moravek MB, Kinnear HM, George J, Batchelor J, Shikanov A, Padmanabhan V, et al. Impact of exogenous testosterone on reproduction in transgender men. Endocrinology. 2020;161(3):bqaa014.
6. Sundaram V, Mok-Lin E. Fertility preservation for the transgender individual. Curr Obstetr Gynecol Rep. 2020;9:1–9.
7. Moravek MB. Fertility preservation options for transgender and gender-nonconforming individuals. Curr Opin Obstet Gynecol. 2019;31(3):170–6.
8. Hembree WC, Cohen-Kettenis PT, Gooren L, Hannema SE, Meyer WJ, Murad MH, et al. Endocrine treatment of gender-dysphoric/gender-incongruent persons: an Endocrine Society clinical practice guideline. J Clin Endocrinol Metab. 2017;102(11):3869–903.
9. De Roo C, Tilleman K, T'Sjoen G, De Sutter P. Fertility options in transgender people. Int Rev Psychiatry. 2016;28(1):112–9.
10. Padmanabhan V, Veiga-Lopez A. Animal models of the polycystic ovary syndrome phenotype. Steroids. 2013;78(8):734–40.
11. Shi D, Vine DF. Animal models of polycystic ovary syndrome: a focused review of rodent models in relationship to clinical phenotypes and cardiometabolic risk. Fertil Steril. 2012;98(1):185–193.e2.
12. Kinnear HM, Constance ES, David A, Marsh EE, Padmanabhan V, Shikanov A, et al. A mouse model to investigate the impact of testosterone therapy on reproduction in transgender men. Hum Reprod. 2019;34(10):2009–17.
13. Ikeda K, Baba T, Noguchi H, Nagasawa K, Endo T, Kiya T, et al. Excessive androgen exposure in female-to-male transsexual persons of reproductive age induces hyperplasia of the ovarian cortex and stroma but not polycystic ovary morphology. Hum Reprod. 2013;28(2):453–61.
14. Futterweit W, Deligdisch L. Histopathological effects of exogenously administered testosterone in 19 female to male transsexuals. J Clin Endocrinol Metab. 1986 Jan;62(1):16–21.
15. Chadha S, Pache TD, Huikeshoven FJM, Brinkmann AO, van derKwast TH. Androgen receptor expression in human ovarian and uterine tissue of long term androgen-treated transsexual women. Hum Pathol. 1994;25(11):1198–204.
16. Grynberg M, Fanchin R, Dubost G, Colau J-C, Brémont-Weil C, Frydman R, et al. Histology of genital tract and breast tissue after long-term testosterone administration in a female-to-male transsexual population. Reprod Biomed Online. 2010;20(4):553–8.
17. Nakamura A, Watanabe M, Sugimoto M, Sako T, Mahmood S, Kaku H, et al. Dose-response analysis of testosterone replacement therapy in patients with female to male gender identity disorder. Endocr J. 2013;60(3):275–81.
18. Steinle K. Hormonal Management of the Female-to-Male Transgender Patient. J Midwifery Womens Health. 2011;56(3):293–302.
19. T'Sjoen G, Van Caenegem E, Wierckx K. Transgenderism and reproduction. Curr Opin Endocrinol Diabetes Obes. 2013;20(6):575–9.
20. Light AD, Obedin-Maliver J, Sevelius JM, Kerns JL. Transgender men who experienced pregnancy after female-to-male gender transitioning. Obstet Gynecol. 2014;124(6):1120–7.

21. Obedin-Maliver J, Makadon HJ. Transgender men and pregnancy. Obstet Med. 2016;9(1):4–8.
22. Light A, Wang L-F, Zeymo A, Gomez-Lobo V. Family planning and contraception use in transgender men. Contraception. 2018;98(4):266–9.
23. La Marca A, Volpe A. Anti-Mullerian hormone (AMH) in female reproduction: is measurement of circulating AMH a useful tool? Clin Endocrinol. 2006;64:603–10.
24. Hansen KR, Hodnett GM, Knowlton N, et al. Correlation of ovarian reserve tests with histologically determined primordial follicle number. Fertil Steril. 2011;95:170–5.
25. Adeleye AJ, Cedars MI, Smith J, Mok-Lin E. Ovarian stimulation for fertility preservation or family building in a cohort of transgender men. J Assist Reprod Genet. 2019;36(10):2155–61.
26. Lee DE, Park SY, Lee SR, Jeong K, Chung HW. Diagnostic usefulness of Transrectal ultrasound compared with transvaginal ultrasound assessment in young Korean women with polycystic ovary syndrome. J Menopausal Med. 2015;21(3):149.
27. Timor-Tritsch IE, Monteagudo A, Rebarber A, Goldstein SR, Tsymbal T. Transrectal scanning: an alternative when transvaginal scanning is not feasible: Transrectal scanning. Ultrasound Obstet Gynecol. 2003;21(5):473–9.
28. Kim S-Y, Kim SK, Lee JR, Woodruff TK. Toward precision medicine for preserving fertility in cancer patients: existing and emerging fertility preservation options for women. J Gynecol Oncol. 2016;27(2):e22.
29. Daar J, Benward J, Collins L, Davis J, Davis O, Francis L, et al. Planned oocyte cryopreservation for women seeking to preserve future reproductive potential: an ethics committee opinion. Fertil Steril. 2018;110(6):1022–8.
30. Wallace SA, Blough KL, Kondapalli LA. Fertility preservation in the transgender patient: expanding oncofertility care beyond cancer. Gynecol Endocrinol. 2014 Dec;30(12):868–71.
31. Maxwell S, Noyes N, Keefe D, Berkeley AS, Goldman KN. Pregnancy outcomes after fertility preservation in transgender men. Obstet Gynecol. 2017;129(6):1031–4.
32. Chen D, Bernardi LA, Pavone ME, Feinberg EC, Moravek MB. Oocyte cryopreservation among transmasculine youth: a case series. J Assist Reprod Genet. 2018;35(11):2057–61.
33. Armuand G, Dhejne C, Olofsson JI, Rodriguez-Wallberg KA. Transgender men's experiences of fertility preservation: a qualitative study. Hum Reprod. 2017;32(2):383–90.
34. Leung A, Sakkas D, Pang S, Thornton K, Resetkova N. Assisted reproductive technology outcomes in female-to-male transgender patients compared with cisgender patients: a new frontier in reproductive medicine. Fertil Steril. 2019;112(5):858–65.
35. Fabregues F, et al. Transdermal testosterone may improve ovarian response to gonadotrophins in low-responder IVF patients: a randomized, clinical trial. Hum Reprod. 2009;24(2):349–59.
36. Cobo A, Garcia-Velasco JA, Domingo J, Remohí J, Pellicer A. Is vitrification of oocytes useful for fertility preservation for age-related fertility decline and in cancer patients? Fertil Steril. 2013;99(6):1485–95.
37. Wierckx K, Elaut E, Van Hoorde B, Heylens G, De Cuypere G, Monstrey S, et al. Sexual desire in trans persons: associations with sex reassignment treatment. J Sex Med. 2014;11(1):107–18.
38. Cho K, et al. Fertility preservation in a transgender man without prolonged discontinuation of testosterone: a case report and literature review. F&S Rep. 2020;1(1):43–7.
39. Gale J, Magee B, Forsyth-Greig A, Visram H, Jackson A. Oocyte cryopreservation in a transgender man on long term testosterone therapy: a case report. F&S Reports. 2021;2:249.
40. Oktay K, Turan V, Bedoschi G, Pacheco FS, Moy F. Fertility preservation success subsequent to concurrent aromatase inhibitor treatment and ovarian stimulation in women with breast cancer. J Clin Oncol. 2015;33(22):2424–9.
41. Wiepjes CM, Nota NM, de Blok CJM, Klaver M, de Vries ALC, Wensing-Kruger SA, et al. The Amsterdam cohort of gender dysphoria study (1972–2015): trends in prevalence, treatment, and regrets. J Sex Med. 2018;15(4):582–90.
42. Heger S, Müller M, Ranke M, Schwarz H-P, Waldhauser F, Partsch C-J, et al. Long-term GnRH agonist treatment for female central precocious puberty does not impair reproductive function. Mol Cell Endocrinol. 2006;254–255:217–20.

43. Linde R, Doelle GC, Alexander N, Kirchner F, Vale W, Rivier J, et al. Reversible inhibition of testicular steroidogenesis and spermatogenesis by a potent gonadotropin-releasing hormone agonist in Normal men: an approach toward the development of a male contraceptive. N Engl J Med. 1981;305(12):663–7.
44. Rothenberg SS, Witchel SF, Menke MN. Oocyte cryopreservation in a transgender male adolescent. N Engl J Med. 2019;380(9):886–7.
45. Insogna IG, Ginsburg E, Srouji S. Fertility preservation for adolescent transgender male patients: a case series. J Adolesc Health. 2020;66:750.
46. Donnez J, Dolmans M, Demylle D, Jadoul P, Pirard C, Squifflet J, et al. Livebirth after orthotopic transplantation of cryopreserved ovarian tissue. Lancet. 2004;364(9443):1405–10.
47. De Roo C, Lierman S, Tilleman K, Peynshaert K, Braeckmans K, Caanen M, et al. Ovarian tissue cryopreservation in female-to-male transgender people: insights into ovarian histology and physiology after prolonged androgen treatment. Reprod Biomed Online. 2017;34(6):557–66.
48. Fasano G, Moffa F, Dechène J, Englert Y, Demeestere I. Vitrification of in vitro matured oocytes collected from antral follicles at the time of ovarian tissue cryopreservation. Reprod Biol Endocrinol. 2011;9(1):150.
49. Segers I, Mateizel I, Van Moer E, Smitz J, Tournaye H, Verheyen G, et al. In vitro maturation (IVM) of oocytes recovered from ovariectomy specimens in the laboratory: a promising "ex vivo" method of oocyte cryopreservation resulting in the first report of an ongoing pregnancy in Europe. J Assist Reprod Genet. 2015;32(8):1221–31.
50. Lierman S, Tilleman K, Braeckmans K, Peynshaert K, Weyers S, T'Sjoen G, et al. Fertility preservation for trans men: frozen-thawed in vitro matured oocytes collected at the time of ovarian tissue processing exhibit normal meiotic spindles. J Assist Reprod Genet. 2017;34(11):1449–56.
51. Telfer EE. Future developments: in vitro growth (IVG) of human ovarian follicles. Acta Obstet Gynecol Scand. 2019;98(5):653–8.
52. Picton HM, Wyns C, Anderson RA, Goossens E, Jahnukainen K, Kliesch S, et al. A European perspective on testicular tissue cryopreservation for fertility preservation in prepubertal and adolescent boys. Hum Reprod. 2015;30(11):2463–75.
53. Chen D, Simons L. Ethical considerations in fertility preservation for transgender youth: a case illustration. Clin Pract Pediatr Psychol. 2018;6(1):93–100.
54. Hudson J, Nahata L, Dietz E, Quinn GP. Fertility counseling for transgender AYAs. Clin Pract Pediatr Psychol. 2018;6(1):84–92.

Chapter 5
Fertility and Fertility Preservation for Transfeminine Adults

Jessica Long, James F. Smith, and Amanda J. Adeleye

Introduction

Certain aspects of gender-affirming treatments such as hormone use or surgery can affect how transgender and nonbinary (TGNB) people are able to conceive. For the majority of individuals assigned male at birth, or born with testicular tissue, sperm are the means by which they are able to contribute to the conception of genetically related children. Medical interventions including the commencement of gender-affirming hormones such as estrogen or anti-androgens, or surgeries like orchiectomy can temporarily or permanently impair the ability to conceive. Many groups including the World Professional Association for Transgender Health, the Endocrine Society, and the American Society for Reproductive Medicine recommend that TGNB individuals be offered fertility preservation prior to starting gender-affirming hormone therapy or proceeding with gender-affirming surgical interventions [1–3]. Fortunately for transfeminine people, there are potentially many ways in which they can conceive biologically related children, but it is important to reflect on the unique challenges that some TGNB people may face when thinking about what options are

---

J. Long
Department of Obstetrics and Gynecology, The University of Chicago, Chicago, IL, USA
e-mail: Jessica.Long@uchospitals.edu

J. F. Smith
Department of Urology; Obstetrics, Gynecology, and Reproductive Sciences; and Health Policy, University of California San Francisco, San Francisco, CA, USA
e-mail: James.smith@ucsf.edu

A. J. Adeleye (✉)
Section of Reproductive Endocrinology and Infertility, Department of Obstetrics and Gynecology, The University of Chicago, Chicago, IL, USA
e-mail: aadeleye@bsd.uchicago.edu

© The Author(s), under exclusive license to Springer Nature Switzerland AG 2023
M. B. Moravek, G. de Haan (eds.), *Reproduction in Transgender and Nonbinary Individuals*, https://doi.org/10.1007/978-3-031-14933-7_5

available. This chapter will review the considerations and interventions for transfeminine people interested in family building to have genetically related children.

Transfeminine People Are Interested in Building Genetically Related Families

Many transfeminine people are interested in having genetically related children. DeSutter et al. surveyed 121 transgender women in the Netherlands, the United Kingdom, Belgium, and France about their history of biological parentage, interest in future family building and fertility preservation. Thirty-nine percent had at least one biological child from a previous relationship. Among the women who had not had children, 40% were interested in having children although the vast majority (90%) did not want to delay gender-affirming treatment to preserve their fertility [4]. In a cross-sectional study of 189 TGNB people in Germany, 69.9% of transfeminine people were interested in having children in the future. Importantly, although the majority of transfeminine people were interested in fertility preservation, only 9.6% of participants had actually preserved gametes [5]. Some transfeminine individuals who are interested in having a genetically related family may have completed their family prior to starting gender-affirming treatments. Tornello et al. explored the pathways to parenthood of 311 TGNB people and found that the majority of transfeminine people who participated in the study had genetically related children that were most often conceived before initiating gender affirmation [6]. It is important to recognize that life stage may influence one's desire to have genetically related children. Multiple studies have demonstrated that adolescents are often uninterested in being a biological parent. Furthermore, an urgency to initiate treatment may influence how adolescents approach fertility preservation [7, 8].

The data are clear that transfeminine people desire to build families before, during, and after their gender affirmation. There appears to be a generational influence to how transfeminine people choose to build their families with individuals who are older at the time of transition potentially having children already. In contrast, younger TGNB individuals may be open to non-biological routes to parenthood. Regardless of age, options for fertility preservation should be readdressed over time as family building goals may change [7].

Obstacles to Family Building

Depending on which gender-affirming options one pursues, transfeminine people may face biological and psychological obstacles to family building. Fortunately, there are a number of advances which may help transfeminine individuals overcome these challenges to become parents.

Biologic Impacts of Gender-Affirming Treatments

There are both nonmedical and medical modalities for gender affirmation that may affect the testes and spermatogenesis.

Tucking is an example of a nonmedical approach to gender affirmation that in some cases may affect testicular function. Tucking refers to the manual movement of the testicles upward into the abdominal cavity. The scrotum allows the testes to exist outside the abdominal cavity in an environment that is typically 4° cooler than the core body temperature. Excessive heat exposure due to the environment or potentially febrile illness, is a known risk factor for abnormal semen parameters [9]. Furthermore, tucking can be associated with orchialgia and in rare cases can lead to testicular torsion. There have been at least two cases described in the literature of transfeminine people who suffered from testicular torsion. In both cases, these women underwent subsequent bilateral orchiectomies [10, 11]. Currently, data are limited on the potential impact of tucking on testicular histology and spermatogenesis. A study from 1985 evaluated tucking as a contraceptive method. After 6 months of daily tucking, the 14 participants had decreased sperm concentrations relative to baseline, ranging from 12 million/ml to 34 million/ml [12].

Transfeminine people may choose to use GnRH agonists/antagonists, estrogen, anti-androgens, or a combination as part of their gender affirmation. The impact of these intervention on the histological architecture of the testes varies. Older studies have suggested a concerning and potentially long-term impact of hormonal therapy on the testes, whereas more recent data suggests that in some cases, the impacts may be less worrisome.

GnRH agonists are also a common component of gender-affirming regimens. GnRH agonists competitively bind to and activate GnRH receptors in the anterior pituitary gland, in turn decreasing FSH and LH production [13]. Downstream, this results in decreased production of testosterone by Leydig cells to castration levels within 2–3 weeks of exposure [14–16]. In the early 1980s, a small number of cisgender men received subcutaneous GnRH agonist that led to 75% of patients having a severe decline in semen parameters. Sexual side effects, specifically an inability to achieve an erection, are also common in cisgender men using GnRH agonists. While these individuals recovered the ability to achieve an erection 2 weeks after stopping subcutaneous GnRH, erection recovery may take longer for patients taking a longer acting GnRH agonist or antagonist. Importantly, complete spermatogenesis was restored 10–14 weeks after the cessation of the GnRH agonist; however, this has not been evaluated systematically in a TGNB population [17].

In a 1977 case series from Riagu et al., orchiectomy specimens were examined after four transfeminine people had used ethinyl estradiol 1–2 mg daily for at least 12 months. On histological examination, testes from all four participants demonstrated significant hyalinization and fibrosis of the seminiferous tubules, the majority of which contained Sertoli cells only [18]. In another cohort of four transfeminine people using ethinyl estradiol, seminiferous tubules again were predominately Sertoli cell only with few spermatogonia. The Sertoli cells also had some unusual features including more lipid like consolidations [19]. Recent trends in gender affirmation therapy utilize estradiol more frequently than ethinyl estradiol. In one of the largest cohorts of transfeminine people reviewed, 108 transfeminine people used varying estrogen therapies in combination with anti-androgens with 0–6 weeks of discontinuation prior to orchiectomy. Histological findings varied significantly with 16.7% of participants with findings of Sertoli cell only seminiferous tubules or tubular shadows. In contrast, complete spermatogenesis was identified in 24.1% of individuals in the study [20]. It is difficult to ascertain the complete impact of gender-affirming hormone therapy due to the varying regimens used, the time during which medications were used, and the time of discontinuation prior to orchiectomy. However, most work in this area demonstrates some negative impact of gender-affirming hormones on testicular histology and spermatogenesis [21].

In addition to potential histologic changes to the testes, there are likely functional impacts to spermatogenesis as the result of exposure to gender-affirming hormones. In a study from Adeleye et al., semen parameters from 28 transfeminine people were assessed. Three groups were compared: women with no history of gender-affirming estrogen, women who had previously used gender-affirming hormones, and women who were currently on hormones at the time of specimen collection. Semen parameters were poor in the group of transfeminine people who used hormones at the time of specimen collection. Importantly, among transfeminine people using hormones at the time of specimen collection, semen parameters ranged from azoospermia to oligospermia with total motile counts that could be used for in vitro fertilization (IVF) and potentially for intrauterine insemination (IUI). There were non-statistically significant differences between transfeminine people who had used estrogen but discontinued prior to specimen collection and those who had never used gender-affirming hormones. The three transfeminine people with a history of gender-affirming hormones who discontinued prior to specimen collection had total motile counts adequate for insemination and penile-vaginal intercourse [22].

Certainly, the surgical absence of either the penis or testes will limit reproductive function. Absence of the penis does not allow for penetrative intercourse although in certain situations, if the testes are retained, sperm could be retrieved surgically. For transfeminine people who have had an orchiectomy, no gametes are available for reproduction. In both cases, transfeminine people who desire genetically related children would ideally cryopreserve sperm prior to surgical intervention. Although there are some interesting preliminary data on in vitro gametogenesis wherein sperm may be generated from stem cells, this work is highly experimental and beyond the scope of this chapter. For more information, readers may appreciate an excellent review from Saitou and Miyauchi [23].

Both medical and surgical modes of gender affirmation may have an impact on future fertility but the degree of the impact may be influenced by the type of affirmation.

Psychological Considerations

Sexual desire and arousal are complex experiences that may be related to gender identity, body image, physical or psychiatric well-being. For transfeminine people, the ability to become aroused and ejaculate are important for either spontaneous conception with penile-vaginal intercourse or for semen collection for assisted reproduction or fertility preservation. The data on potential psychological or performance related barriers to reproduction for transfeminine people are limited. However, available data support that transfeminine individuals have multifactorial inputs that may affect their ability to become aroused, similar to cisgender women. It is important to recognize that psychological limitations to arousal and ejaculation are not all encompassing and some transfeminine people have no issues in this area. Nahata et al. surveyed 78 TGNB adolescents and noted that a minority of transgender young women (1.4%) stated discomfort with masturbation as a reason that they deferred fertility preservation. More common reasons for deferring fertility preservation in this adolescent group included a lack of interest in family building, a desire to adopt, or concerns about costs [24].

Among adult cisgender women, several studies have demonstrated potential challenges with sexual arousal or function. In a cross-sectional survey of 214 transfeminine people using gender-affirming hormones, 62.4% of participants reported a decrease in sexual desire after the initiation of gender-affirming medical treatments. Importantly, transfeminine people who had undergone vaginoplasty reported an increase in sexual desire [25]. In a longitudinal study of 53 transfeminine individuals using gender-affirming hormones, the majority experienced a decrease in sex drive over the year of the study [26].

Some studies have demonstrated a relationship between serum testosterone and estrogen levels with sexual desire and function, whereas others have not. Bettocchi et al. administered the International index of Erectile Function (IIEF-15) questionnaire to 25 transfeminine people, assessed penile function with penile color-coded Doppler ultrasonography with pharmacological stimulation and finally examined nocturnal penile tumescence episodes. IIEF scores and Doppler ultrasonography were not associated with testosterone levels; however, nocturnal penile tumescence was associated with testosterone levels [27]. Greenstein et al. demonstrated preserved erectile function in four presumably cisgender men who were medically or surgically castrated for prostate cancer. They also demonstrated that there was an association between serum testosterone levels and the ability to achieve an erection with visual stimulation [28].

There are several reasons why a transfeminine individual may or may not be able to become aroused and ejaculate for procreative purposes. For more information on the sexual function of transfeminine people, see Chap. 9 on "non-procreative reproductive issues and sexual function in transfeminine individuals."

Partner Considerations

Ultimately, the ability to reproduce depends upon having available oocytes, sperm, an environment for conception, and a uterus to carry a pregnancy, regardless of gender. Transfeminine people may face unique challenges to family building depending on who they chose to partner with or if they choose to partner with anyone at all.

Transfeminine individuals may have a partner who does not have ovaries, a uterus, or both. In this case, the couple may require either an oocyte donor or possibly a gestational carrier. Transfeminine people who are single would need an oocyte donor and gestational carrier for assistance with family building.

Fertility Preservation Options

Reasons to Cryopreserve Sperm

Transfeminine people may wish to cryopreserve sperm for a number of reasons. Some may wish to cryopreserve sperm before initiating gender-affirming treatments or prior to surgical affirmation. Others may have already sought medical gender affirmation but with increasing education about fertility, would like to preserve sperm before continuing or advancing their gender affirmation. Yet another group may know that their family building goals will involve the use of assisted reproductive technology based upon their sexual orientation thus, regardless of their gender affirmation plans, preserving sperm for a time when they are ready to family build is a sensible option.

Methods for Sperm Collection

There are several methods through which sperm can be cryopreserved. Techniques include cryopreservation of semen through spontaneous ejaculation, electroejaculation, or the surgical retrieval of sperm. The latter two techniques require the assistance of a reproductive urologist.

The most common method for cryopreserving sperm is via ejaculation and semen cryopreservation. This method has been widely used in other settings including at donor sperm banks or for people undergoing gonadotoxic treatments for a cancer diagnosis. Transfeminine people may produce a semen sample via ejaculation, typically at a sperm bank but depending on the storage facility they may produce in a private setting as well. People that do not plan to use their sperm with an intimate partner or are unsure should follow regulatory guidelines for the use of sperm with a third party. This may include a physical exam and a series of sexually transmitted infectious disease panels.

5 Fertility and Fertility Preservation for Transfeminine Adults

Some transfeminine people may not be able to experience erections or ejaculate; in this case additional stimulation may be helpful. One approach to induce ejaculation is with penile vibratory stimulation. Ejaculation may be accomplished by stimulating the dorsal penile nerve using a medical vibrator with a frequency of approximately 100 Hz at the base of the glans penis [29]. In a study of 211 presumably cisgender men (patients referred to as men) with neurogenic injuries limiting ejaculation, 89% of these men achieved ejaculation within 2 min of high frequency stimulation [30]. Importantly, penile vibratory stimulation can result in skin abrasions which should be monitored during and after the procedure.

For transfeminine people who are unable to produce a semen sample, rectal electrical stimulation may be considered. Electroejaculation generally requires anesthesia for people with intact pelvic sensation. Under the care of a urologist, rectoscopy to evaluate for rectal trauma and instillation of pH appropriate media into the bladder are advisable prior to treatment. Rectal electrical stimulation is applied typically at 2.5–3.0 V for brief periods of time until ejaculate is produced. This continues until no further ejaculate is identified. Retroejaculation is common with this technique. At the end of the case, the bladder is catheterized to retrieve any additional sperm [29].

In a large series of 500 cisgender men with spinal cord injuries, Brackett et al. reviewed the semen parameters after masturbation, penile vibratory stimulation, or electroejaculation. Sixty-three percent of specimens in this study had a total motile count exceeding five million which as a fresh sample could be adequate for intrauterine insemination and certainly for in vitro fertilization (IVF) [31]. Data on penile vibratory stimulation and electroejaculation are limited in the transfeminine population. The primary advantage of electroejaculation over surgical sperm retrieval is the potential for obtaining enough sperm from one procedure for multiple intrauterine insemination procedures. While no incision is necessary with this technique, it does require general anesthesia for a patient with intact sensation, adding significant logistical and cost barriers. Furthermore, the equipment needed for the technique is not widely available.

Transfeminine people who find ejaculation of any sort to be intolerable or who do not have a functional penis may opt for surgical retrieval of sperm. In some cases, transfeminine people may undergo percutaneous epididymal sperm aspiration (PESA) whereby sperm are retrieved via aspiration from the epididymis or testicular sperm aspiration (TESA) under local anesthesia. More invasive procedures exist including testicular sperm extraction (TESE) and microsurgical epididymal sperm aspiration (MESA). TESE procedures involve an incision into the testicles, biopsies are collected, and sperm are identified from the seminiferous tubules and surrounding tissue. In a MESA procedure, an incision is made into the epididymis and with the assistance of a microscope, fluid is aspirated from the proximal epididymal tubules. Intracytoplasmic sperm injection (ICSI) is indicated after these procedures. Interestingly, in cisgender men with obstructive azoospermia, MESA-ICSI has been associated with higher pregnancy rates compared to TESE-ICSI [32]. These techniques are more widely available and can be performed wherever a reproductive urologist is available.

Importantly, for transfeminine people seeking orchiectomy, it is possible to retrieve sperm at the time of surgery (Personal Communication: James Smith, MD MS). However, the presence of sperm in the surgical specimen may depend on whether an individual completed gender-affirming hormone therapy prior to surgery. Sperm have been successfully retrieved and used for pregnancy from azoospermic cisgender men undergoing orchiectomy for testicular cancer [33]. Success with this technique for transfeminine people has yet to be defined systematically.

The quantity of sperm needed for assisted reproduction varies. It is important to consider that typically half of the sperm frozen will thaw successfully [34]. When intrauterine insemination is used, pregnancy rates are more likely when the post-wash specimen is over five million [35]. In contrast, just hundreds to thousands of sperm are needed for IVF, particularly with intracytoplasmic sperm injection. Many other factors should be considered when thinking about the quantity of sperm required for conception. Transfeminine people contemplating fertility preservation should consider the factors that their partner may contribute including age and any underlying infertility. In general, patients with at least ten million moving sperm in their ejaculate could use this sample for 1 IUI or multiple IVF cycles. Each ejaculate can be divided into multiple aliquots.

Other Considerations for Sperm Cryopreservation

Live births have been achieved with sperm cryopreserved for over 40 years and it is possible that sperm could be stored indefinitely in liquid nitrogen [36]. For some, long-term storage of sperm may introduce socioeconomic and ethical complexities. In particular, adolescents storing sperm may be faced with several years of storage fees and may ultimately decide not to have genetically related children. In addition, several years of storage fees can prove to be a financial hardship for a population that is often economically disadvantaged [37].

As with any individual cryopreserving gametes, transfeminine people must consider the disposition of their sperm in the event of their death or incapacitation. Questions surrounding whether or not an individual would want to be a genetic parent after their death and with whom they could conceive in these situations are critically important to consider prior to cryopreservation.

Accessibility to fertility preservation may be challenging for some TGNB individuals. Adequate counseling about fertility preservation and facilities to collect and store sperm are not readily available in all settings. Urologic surgeons with expertise and awareness of the needs of transfeminine people may be an even more scarce resource when they need procedural interventions. Transfeminine people that have physical access to facilities and specialists may still be limited by economic circumstances. Unfortunately, few countries have made progress towards mandating fertility preservation coverage for TGNB individuals.

Assisted Reproduction

For transfeminine people interested in having genetically related children, a wide variety of family building options may be available. Options are dependent on both personal choice and what biological resources a person has when they want to conceive. Assisted reproductive treatments may be helpful for transfeminine people who would like to grow their families but are unable to participate in penile-vaginal intercourse. For transfeminine people in need of reproductive assistance, current options include intrauterine insemination and in vitro fertilization (IVF) with a partner with a uterus or with a gestational carrier.

Intrauterine Insemination

Intrauterine insemination is a process by which sperm are placed in the uterine cavity at the time of anticipated ovulation. The recipient with a uterus either ovulates regularly or can be induced to ovulate with medication. Ovulation occurs from follicles which are structures within the ovary that contain layers of granulosa cells surrounding a single oocyte. Follicles typically undergo atresia but during a menstrual cycle one follicle is selected to mature and releases an oocyte that may be fertilized in the fallopian tube. Under hormonal stimulation, multiple follicles can be induced to grow and potentially release oocytes.

The person undergoing ovarian stimulation may be monitored with a pelvic ultrasound to assess follicular growth. Alternatively, an ovulation predictor kit may be used to detect a luteinizing hormone surge. At the time of anticipated ovulation, sperm may be placed in the vagina with a syringe, the cervix via a cervical cap, or into the uterus using a flexible intrauterine catheter passed through the cervical canal. Intrauterine insemination is associated with the highest pregnancy rates [38]. For transfeminine people who are able to produce semen, fresh sperm can be used. Otherwise, previously cryopreserved sperm prepared for insemination may be used. For intrauterine insemination, after processing, a minimum of five to ten million sperm are recommended [39].

In Vitro Fertilization

In vitro fertilization (IVF) is a process wherein oocytes are fertilized with sperm in the lab. To accomplish this, a person with ovaries undergoes ovarian stimulation to rescue maturing follicles selected in a given cycle. As opposed to ovulation induction or superovulation for insemination where the goal is to stimulate the growth of 1–3 follicles, ovarian stimulation for IVF aims to grow several or all of the larger follicles in a given cycle. A uterus is not necessary for ovarian stimulation but if there is no uterus, the couple will need a gestational carrier, also known as a surrogate. Alternatively, a transfeminine individual may work with an oocyte donor who will undergo ovarian stimulation and donate their eggs for conception.

During ovarian stimulation for IVF, follicles are induced to grow with the use of daily subcutaneous gonadotropin injections. The ovaries are monitored regularly for follicular growth with pelvic ultrasounds, estradiol levels, and at times progesterone or other hormone levels. The goal of ovarian stimulation for IVF is to grow a cohort of large follicles in a synchronous fashion. Larger follicles are associated with a higher likelihood of having a mature oocyte at retrieval. When lead follicles are typically 18–20 mm in size, final maturation of the follicles is triggered with a medication with LH activity such as human chorionic gonadotropin or a GnRH agonist. Approximately 36 h later, oocytes are retrieved via ultrasound guided transvaginal aspiration of follicular fluid. This procedure often occurs under monitored anesthesia care. In the case of transfeminine people, they may provide sperm that day or thaw sperm that were previously frozen for fertility preservation. Normally fertilized oocytes (embryos) are cultured for 3–6 days. One or more surviving embryos are transferred to the uterus of the partner or gestational carrier with a speculum guided pelvic exam and passage of a transcervical catheter to the intrauterine cavity. Any additional embryos can be cryopreserved for future use. Alternatively, all embryos may be frozen if genetic testing for aneuploidy or a specific monosomic genetic mutation testing if desired.

There are many factors that determine the success of an IVF cycle including age of the person contributing oocytes, sperm quality, and potentially any underlying infertility issues. Outcomes from assisted reproduction for TGNB people are limited but promising. Discussion and management of IVF should be completed with the assistance of a reproductive endocrinologist.

Family Building Options for Transfeminine People

How a transfeminine person builds a genetically related family will depend on whether or not they are in a relationship with someone (and if not, desire to parent without a partner), what gametes are available, and whether or not a partner has a uterus and ovaries. Additionally, the psychological well-being that a transfeminine individual and their potential partner have during this process is key. As an example, although they may have a penis and testes, they may not tolerate ejaculation or penile-vaginal intercourse. Fortunately, many opportunities for assisted reproduction are available to transfeminine people that are described in this section.

Approach for Transfeminine People with Testes, a Penis, and the Ability to Ejaculate (Table 5.1)

Transfeminine people who currently have testes, a penis, and the ability to ejaculate have multiple conception options which depend in part on their partner, if partnered. They may be able to conceive with penetrative penile-vaginal intercourse or use

Table 5.1 Excludes traditional surrogacy where a person with a uterus and ovaries is inseminated via intrauterine insemination to carry a pregnancy for an intended parent

		Partner gender				
	Mode of conception	Single	Cisgender female	Transmasculine person	Cisgender male	Transfeminine person
Transfeminine person	Spontaneous conception/ intercourse		+	+		
	Intrauterine Insemination		+	+		
	IVF		+	+		
	IVF with GC	+ (with donor oocyte)	*If medically necessary	+	+ (with donor oocyte)	+ (with donor oocyte)

Options depend on the availability and quantity of sperm and possibly presence of a penis and ability to ejaculate

IVF = in vitro fertilization, *GC* = Gestational carrier

various assisted reproductive technologies such as intrauterine insemination or in vitro fertilization. Oocytes could be derived autologously if the partner has ovaries or they could use donor oocytes. If their partner does not have a uterus or does not want to carry the pregnancy, they could consider use of a gestational carrier.

Approach for Transfeminine People Who Do Not Have Testes or a Penis but Cryopreserved Sperm (Table 5.1)

When a transfeminine person does not have testes but cryopreserved sperm in advance, options remain for conception. If the partner has a uterus and ovaries, all assisted reproductive options may be available depending on how much sperm was cryopreserved. Generally, sperm cryopreserved from ejaculate may be used for insemination, whereas surgically retrieved sperm requires IVF. Whether or not donor oocytes or a gestational carrier is needed would depend on the partner.

Approach for the Single Transfeminine Individual (Table 5.1)

As long as sperm are available—either fresh or cryopreserved, single transfeminine people could conceive using IVF with an oocyte donor and gestational carrier. Notably, working with an oocyte donor and gestational carrier may be associated with some economic and legal hurdles. Transfeminine people who opt to use a gestational carrier should be aware that the legality of gestational surrogacy varies by location. There is an increasing interest in uterine transplant as a means for transfeminine people to carry a pregnancy however to date, this technique has been used in cisgender women who typically have a congenital absence of the uterus [40]. These transplants are performed at select settings globally and to date have not been performed for transfeminine people.

Success Rates with Reproductive Options for Transfeminine People

Success rates with assisted reproduction vary depending on characteristics of the transfeminine individual, as well as the person contributing oocytes and a uterus. Transfeminine people without a history of hormone therapy may be able to produce normal semen specimens [22]. Should they partner with someone who has a uterus and ovaries, it is conceivable that fecundity could range from 15 to 33% per cycle depending on the frequency of intercourse [41]. For people pursuing IVF in the United States in 2018, the live birth rate per IVF cycle when the person undergoing ovarian stimulation was under 35 was 47.6%.

Conclusion

Transfeminine people have the ability to have genetically related children. Certain gender-affirming treatments can influence their success with conception. A thoughtful discussion about family building goals and gender affirmation may identify individuals who would benefit from fertility preservation. Ultimately transfeminine people may have many options for conception that depend on the gametes available and whether or not a uterus is available to carry the pregnancy.

References

1. Coleman E, Bockting W, Botzer M, Cohen-Kettenis P, DeCuypere G, Feldman J, et al. Standards of care for the health of transsexual, transgender, and gender-nonconforming people, version 7. Int J Transgenderism. 2012;13(4):165–232.
2. Hembree WC, Cohen-Kettenis PT, Gooren L, Hannema SE, Meyer WJ, Murad MH, et al. Endocrine treatment of gender-dysphoric/gender-incongruent persons: an endocrine society* clinical practice guideline. J Clin Endocrinol Metab. 2017 [cited 2017 Oct 23]; Available from http://academic.oup.com/jcem/article/doi/10.1210/jc.2017-01658/4157558/Endocrine-Treatment-of
3. Ethics Committee of the American Society for Reproductive Medicine. Access to fertility services by transgender persons: an Ethics Committee opinion. Fertil Steril. 2015;104(5):1111–5.
4. De Sutter P, Kira K, Verschoor A, Hotimsky A. The desire to have children and the preservation of fertility in transsexual women: a survey. Int J Transgenderism. 2002;6(3):215–21.
5. Auer MK, Fuss J, Nieder TO, Briken P, Biedermann SV, Stalla GK, et al. Desire to have children among transgender people in Germany: a cross-sectional multi-center study. J Sex Med. 2018;15(5):757–67.
6. Tornello SL, Riskind RG, Babić A. Transgender and gender non-binary parents' pathways to parenthood. Psychol Sex Orientat Gend Divers. 2019;6(2):232–41.
7. Morrison A, Olezeski C, Cron J, Kallen AN. A pilot study to assess attitudes toward future fertility and parenthood in transgender and gender expansive adolescents. Transgender Health. 2020;5(2):129–37.
8. Strang JF, Jarin J, Call D, Clark B, Wallace GL, Anthony LG, et al. Transgender youth fertility attitudes questionnaire: measure development in nonautistic and autistic transgender youth and their parents. J Adolesc Health 2017 [cited 2017 Dec 13]; Available from http://linkinghub.elsevier.com/retrieve/pii/S1054139X17304056
9. Abdelhamid MHM, Esquerre-Lamare C, Walschaerts M, Ahmad G, Mieusset R, Hamdi S, et al. Experimental mild increase in testicular temperature has drastic, but reversible, effect on sperm aneuploidy in men: a pilot study. Reprod Biol. 2019 Jun;19(2):189–94.
10. Debarbo CJM. Rare cause of testicular torsion in a transwoman: a case report. Urol Case Rep. 2020;33:101422.
11. Epps T, McCormick B, Ali A, Duboy A, Gillen J, Martinez D, et al. From tucking to twisting; A case of self-induced testicular torsion in a cross dressing male. Urol Case Rep. 2016;7:51–2.
12. Mieusset R, Grandjean H, Mansat A, Pontonnier F. Inhibiting effect of artificial cryptorchidism on spermatogenesis. Fertil Steril. 1985;43(4):589–94.
13. Mattawanon N, Spencer JB, Schirmer DA, Tangpricha V. Fertility preservation options in transgender people: a review. Rev Endocr Metab Disord. 2018 Sep;19(3):231–42.
14. Labrie F, Cusan L, Séguin C, Bélanger A, Pelletier G, Reeves J, et al. Antifertility effects of LHRH agonists in the male rat and inhibition of testicular steroidogenesis in man. Int J Fertil. 1980;25(3):157–70.

15. Labrie F, Bélanger A, Luu-The V, Labrie C, Simard J, Cusan L, et al. Gonadotropin-releasing hormone agonists in the treatment of prostate cancer. Endocr Rev. 2005;26(3):361–79.
16. Lunglmayr G, Girsch E, Meixner EM, Viehberger G, Bieglmayer C. Effects of long term GnRH analogue treatment on hormone levels and spermatogenesis in patients with carcinoma of the prostate. Urol Res. 1988;16(4):315–9.
17. Linde R, Doelle GC, Alexander N, Kirchner F, Vale W, Rivier J, et al. Reversible inhibition of testicular steroidogenesis and spermatogenesis by a potent gonadotropin-releasing hormone agonist in normal men: an approach toward the development of a male contraceptive. N Engl J Med. 1981;305(12):663–7.
18. Rodriguez-Rigau LJ, Tcholakian RK, Smith KD, Steinberger E. In vitro steroid metabolic studies in human testes I: effects of estrogen on progesterone metabolism. Steroids. 1977;29(6):771–86.
19. Lu CC, Steinberger A. Effects of estrogen on human seminiferous tubules: light and electron microscopic analysis. Am J Anat. 1978;153(1):1–13.
20. Schneider F, Neuhaus N, Wistuba J, Zitzmann M, Heß J, Mahler D, et al. Testicular functions and clinical characterization of patients with gender dysphoria (GD) undergoing sex reassignment surgery (SRS). J Sex Med. 2015;12(11):2190–200.
21. Schneider F, Kliesch S, Schlatt S, Neuhaus N. Andrology of male-to-female transsexuals: influence of cross-sex hormone therapy on testicular function. Andrology. 2017;5(5):873–80.
22. Adeleye AJ, Reid G, Kao C-N, Mok-Lin E, Smith JF. Semen parameters among transgender women with a history of hormonal treatment. Urology 2018 Oct [cited 2018 Dec 19]; Available from https://linkinghub.elsevier.com/retrieve/pii/S0090429518310872
23. Saitou M, Miyauchi H. Gametogenesis from pluripotent stem cells. Cell Stem Cell. 2016;18(6):721–35.
24. Nahata L, Tishelman AC, Caltabellotta NM, Quinn GP. Low fertility preservation utilization among transgender youth. J Adolesc Health. 2017;61(1):40–4.
25. Wierckx K, Elaut E, Van Hoorde B, Heylens G, De Cuypere G, Monstrey S, et al. Sexual desire in trans persons: associations with sex reassignment treatment. J Sex Med. 2014;11(1):107–18.
26. Wierckx K, Van Caenegem E, Schreiner T, Haraldsen I, Fisher AD, Fisher A, et al. Cross-sex hormone therapy in trans persons is safe and effective at short-time follow-up: results from the European network for the investigation of gender incongruence. J Sex Med. 2014;11(8):1999–2011.
27. Bettocchi C, Palumbo F, Cormio L, Ditonno P, Battaglia M, Selvaggi FP. The effects of androgen depletion on human erectile function: a prospective study in male-to-female transsexuals. Int J Impot Res. 2004 Dec;16(6):544–6.
28. Greenstein A, Plymate SR, Katz PG. Visually stimulated erection in castrated men. J Urol. 1995;153(3 Pt 1):650–2.
29. Fode M, Ohl DA, Sønksen J. A step-wise approach to sperm retrieval in men with neurogenic anejaculation. Nat Rev Urol. 2015;12(11):607–16.
30. Brackett NL, Ferrell SM, Aballa TC, Amador MJ, Padron OF, Sonksen J, et al. An analysis of 653 trials of penile vibratory stimulation in men with spinal cord injury. J Urol. 1998;159(6):1931–4.
31. Brackett NL, Ibrahim E, Iremashvili V, Aballa TC, Lynne CM. Treatment for ejaculatory dysfunction in men with spinal cord injury: an 18-year single center experience. J Urol. 2010;183(6):2304–8.
32. van Wely M, Barbey N, Meissner A, Repping S, Silber SJ. Live birth rates after MESA or TESE in men with obstructive azoospermia: is there a difference? Hum Reprod. 2015;30(4):761–6.
33. Baniel J, Sella A. Sperm extraction at orchiectomy for testis cancer. Fertil Steril. 2001;75(2):260–2.
34. O'Connell M, McClure N, Lewis SEM. The effects of cryopreservation on sperm morphology, motility and mitochondrial function. Hum Reprod. 2002;17(3):704–9.
35. van Weert J-M, Repping S, Van Voorhis BJ, van der Veen F, Bossuyt PMM, Mol BWJ. Performance of the postwash total motile sperm count as a predictor of pregnancy at the time of intrauterine insemination: a meta-analysis. Fertil Steril. 2004;82(3):612–20.

36. Szell AZ, Bierbaum RC, Hazelrigg WB, Chetkowski RJ. Live births from frozen human semen stored for 40 years. J Assist Reprod Genet. 2013;30(6):743–4.
37. Carpenter CS, Eppink ST, Gonzales G. Transgender status, gender identity, and socioeconomic outcomes in the United States. ILR Rev. 2020;73(3):573–99.
38. Carroll N, Palmer JR. A comparison of intrauterine versus intracervical insemination in fertile single women. Fertil Steril. 2001;75(4):656–60.
39. Schlegel PN, Sigman M, Collura B, De Jonge CJ, Eisenberg ML, Lamb DJ, et al. Diagnosis and treatment of infertility in men: AUA/ASRM guideline part I. J Urol. 2021;205(1):36–43.
40. Jones BP, Saso S, Bracewell-Milnes T, Thum M-Y, Nicopoullos J, Diaz-Garcia C, et al. Human uterine transplantation: a review of outcomes from the first 45 cases. BJOG Int J Obstet Gynaecol. 2019;126(11):1310–9.
41. Pfeifer S, Butts S, Fossum G, Gracia C, La Barbera A, Mersereau J, et al. Optimizing natural fertility: a committee opinion. Fertil Steril. 2017;107(1):52–8.

Chapter 6
Obstetric, Antenatal, and Postpartum Care for Transgender and Nonbinary People

Gnendy Indig, Sebastian Ramos, and Daphna Stroumsa

Introduction

The OB turned out to be lovely, actually trans competent, and queer. He was less interested than my midwife was in me having a C-section, willing to let me stay pregnant longer, better at informed consent, and a far better listener. By the end of my first visit with the OB, I liked him better than the midwife, trusted him more, and felt better supported … Everyone I knew had prepared me to love midwives and be cautious around OBs—meeting Mark Yudln was my first lesson in specificity. Who your care providers are matters far more than their role or professional training.—J Wallace Skelton, Baby Escape Plan Two, Remedy [1]

For many transgender and nonbinary (TGNB) people, the word "family" extends well beyond, and at times excludes biological ties. Kinship refers to the pattern of social relationships that form families and communities. Classically, anthropologists have thought of Western kinship as ties based on biological or legal constructs [2]. Kathy Weston diverged from that framework when she described the concept of queer kinship in her book "Families we Choose." She describes how queer people form their own "chosen families," often due to being ostracized from their biological families, and form communities around those relationships [3]. Later scholarly work expands on how queer kinship allows for sexual and gender minorities to lean on

---

G. Indig
Department of Obstetrics and Gynecology, University of Michigan Medical School, University of Vermont Medical Center, Burlington, VT, USA
e-mail: gnendy.indig@uvmhealth.org

S. Ramos
Department of Obstetrics and Gynecology, Maternal Fetal Medicine, Women and Infant Hospital, Providence, RI, USA
e-mail: seramos@wihri.org

D. Stroumsa (✉)
Department of Obstetrics and Gynecology, Michigan Medicine, Ann Arbor, MI, USA
e-mail: daphnast@med.umich.edu

© The Author(s), under exclusive license to Springer Nature Switzerland AG 2023
M. B. Moravek, G. de Haan (eds.), *Reproduction in Transgender and Nonbinary Individuals*, https://doi.org/10.1007/978-3-031-14933-7_6

each other for care during illness and in health [4]. Thus, when TGNB people expand their families, their support structure might look differently than cisgender individuals. Additionally, societal expectations and ideals around biological families might be emotionally loaded and contribute to stress around pregnancy and childbirth.

While it is the case that, biologically or otherwise, TGNB people have been creating families and kin for a long time, there is a recent increase in research on pregnancies carried by transmasculine people and the way they build their families. The majority of the data are not population-based, but there is an increasing number of qualitative studies and small case-series focused on transgender pregnancies. Data from the PRIDE Study, a longitudinal cohort study of LGBTQ+ people surveyed 1694 transgender and gender-expansive people and found 210 respondents who have been pregnant with a total of 433 pregnancies in that cohort [5]. While data from these studies continues to increase, there is still scant data on how healthcare providers should care for transmasculine people during these pregnancies.

In this chapter we explore the existing data regarding pregnancy in TGNB people, spanning from preconception care to lactation. The majority of this chapter will deal with pregnancy in transmasculine people. We will briefly touch on lactation in transfeminine individuals as well.

Guiding Principles of Care

For many TGNB people, accessing and receiving healthcare can be a highly traumatizing event. Prior negative healthcare experience and gender minority stress both contribute to the anxiety and avoidance around accessing healthcare.

Prior Negative Healthcare Experiences

The 2015 US transgender survey (USTS), the largest survey of transgender people with 27,715 respondents, found that 33% of transgender people had a negative experience in healthcare directly related to their transgender status and that 23% avoided seeing the doctor when they needed to because of fear of being mistreated as a transgender person. That survey found that only 6% of providers knew "almost everything" or "most things" about caring for transgender people [6]. Obstetrics and Gynecology clinics can be particularly dysphoric for transmasculine people because of how gendered the environment and language used can be. In a small qualitative study ($n = 8$) of pregnancy in transmasculine people, all participants shared that none of their providers were experts in transgender care, and most participants reported issues with gendered language during their appointments [7].

To address this, clinics should consider making changes to be more inclusive of TGNB patients [8]. Some language-specific recommendations include: using the term "sexual and reproductive health" instead of "women's health" on clinic signage and forms. Intake forms should include options for transgender and nonbinary gender identity and should ask about preferred terminology for anatomy. In a randomized controlled trial of perinatal healthcare providers, a 40-min education session around transgender pregnancy care increased provider knowledge on transgender topics, decreased misconceptions and prejudice towards LGBTQ patients, increased use of appropriate language, and decreased heteronormative attitudes around pregnancy and birth [9]. Such educational opportunities should be implemented in reproductive health clinics along with transitions to non-gendered signage and intake forms.

Minority Stress

Minority stress framework refers to the phenomenon that discrimination, marginalization, and stress of minorities adversely affect their health. Gender-related minority stress results from increased stigma and discrimination that transgender people face in society and in healthcare, which leads to adverse overall health outcomes, mental health effects, and subsequent increased substance use [10, 11]. Cisnormativity in society and especially in pregnancy adds an additional layer of stress to the pregnancy of transmasculine patients. Providers need to account for this with both support and institutional changes.

Malmquist et al. explored how minority stress impacts pregnancy in lesbian, bisexual, and transgender (LBT) patients via a qualitative study. They conducted 13 semi-structured interviews with 17 participants. They found that cisnormativity around pregnancy and past homophobic/transphobic experience in healthcare increases the anxiety and fear of childbirth and insufficient care in LBT patients. The respondents expressed being on the receiving end of hetero- and cisnormative assumptions and how such experiences lead to hypervigilance when interacting within the healthcare system [12]. That hypervigilance is well-founded, as misclassification based on gender identity can lead to disastrous outcomes. Stroumsa et al. reported a case where a 32-year man with abdominal pain presented to the ED. He reported that he was a transgender man and that he had a positive pregnancy test at home but he was misclassified as a man with abdominal pain. It was only several hours later, when he was re-evaluated that the possibility of pregnancy was considered on the differential for abdominal pain. Bedside US confirmed an advanced pregnancy with unclear presence of fetal cardiac activity. Physical exam demonstrated a gravid abdomen, a dilated cervix, and cord prolapse. Fetal cardiac activity was absent and he delivered a stillborn infant [13]. This case highlights how gender-based discrimination can have disastrous outcomes.

Gender minority stress is additionally compounded by intersectional identities like race and ethnicity. Minority stress of BIPOC (Black, Indigenous, People of Color) people adds additional layers of adverse health and perinatal outcomes. Multiple studies have demonstrated that stress by experiencing and/or exposure to racism is associated with poorer health outcomes and adverse birth outcomes [14].

Trauma-Informed Care

When caring for any patient, providers should be aware of how prior trauma can affect both the health of their patients and the care they provide. Trauma-informed care requires recognition of the trauma TGNB people face in society and in healthcare, and the interventions they might require to address and deliver their healthcare. TGNB people are disproportionately affected by trauma, including transphobia, structural racism, housing, food insecurity, physical and sexual abuse, and child abuse [15]. They are also more likely to experience adverse childhood experiences [16], predisposing them to substance use and suicidality [17]. The disproportional rate at which TGNB people experience traumatic events requires providers to ensure that they practice trauma-informed care. The Substance Abuse and Mental Health Services Administration (SAMHSA) outlines the 6 components of trauma-informed care. (1) Safety: creating a safe physical space. (2) Trustworthiness and Transparency: institutions should be transparent about their operations and decisions. (3) Peer Support: connect trauma survivors with other survivors. (4) Collaboration and Mutuality: true partnering and leveling of power differences between staff and clients. (5) Empowerment, Voice, and Choice: recognizing and building up the individual's strength and experience. (6) Cultural, Historical, and Gender Issues: organization actively moves past cultural stereotypes and biases [18]. Providers should ensure that they and their staff are practicing trauma-informed care with all their patients to improve the health and healthcare delivery of trauma survivors.

Language

TGNB patients should be asked on their first prenatal visit how they refer to their anatomy, themselves, their pregnancy, and their support people. Their responses should be documented in the medical record for later encounters. While some people may choose to use standard terminology like vagina, uterus, etc., others might prefer alternative terms that are not loaded with gendered meaning or use terminology typically associated with masculinity, such as front hole, mangina, reproductive organs, etc. Intake forms and initial history should explicitly ask about appropriate terminology so it can be used consistently in the patient's care and charting.

Summary Guiding principles in caring for transmasculine patients and their pregnancies involves awareness around how minority stress can impact the health of their patient. Providers should ensure that they practice trauma-informed care to reduce the psychosocial impact of healthcare on trauma survivors. Providers, clinic signage, and forms should be gender neutral, inclusive of all genders, and ask about specific needs surrounding terminology and language.

Abortion Care

Moseson et al. found that 54% (233/433) of pregnancies in transmasculine patients are unplanned and that 11% of respondents felt that they are at risk for unintended pregnancy [5]. Pregnant people should always be asked whether their pregnancies are planned and/or desired. TGNB people, like their cisgender counterparts, should be counseled about their pregnancy options and have access to abortion care. Current estimates state that 18% of pregnancies in 2017 ended in abortion [19]. Jones et al. sought to estimate the number of abortions in transgender and gender nonconforming individuals. They examined data from the Guttmacher Institute's 2017 Abortion Provider Consensus, which surveyed all abortion-providing facilities in the USA. They estimated that clinics performed between 462 and 530 abortions for transmasculine and nonbinary patients. Of these, 23% of clinics provided trans-specific care [20]. That data tells us that transgender and gender nonconforming individuals access and need abortion services.

Abortion methods include medication and procedural options. In 2017, 39% of all abortions were through medications [19]. Moseson et al. sought to investigate the experience and preferences around abortion in transgender and gender nonconforming individuals. Among the 1694 eligible survey respondents, 433 lifetime pregnancies were reported with 92 abortions. Of those, 45% underwent a medication abortion and 41% underwent a surgical abortion. All respondents were asked what abortion method they would prefer if they would require one. They found that 42% would prefer medication abortion, 13% would prefer surgical, and 30% didn't know. In practice, 89% of those who said they prefer surgical, underwent a surgical abortion while only 50% of those who stated they would choose medication abortion eventually underwent medication abortion. One reason for the discrepancy is the legal gestational limits on medication abortion. Preferences for either method were asked in this survey as well. Reasons for medication abortion included being less invasive, increased privacy, and less anesthesia. Reasons to prefer surgical abortion included faster time to expulsion, less pain, and no need for hormones. Respondents who reported a pregnancy that ended in abortion were also asked about gender-related recommendations to improve the abortion experience. Responses included gender-neutral intake forms and language, increasing availability of gender-affirming abortion care, and increased patient privacy [21].

Regardless of the preferred method, transmasculine individuals evidently need and use abortion services. Clinics and providers who provide abortion services should make sure that their staff is trained in providing appropriate care to patients of all genders.

Preconception

Caring for all pregnant people should ideally start prior to conception with preconception counseling and screening. While most preconception care for transmasculine patients will be similar to care received by cisgender women, several unique issues arise. While we don't have data on the rates of adequate preconception care in transmasculine people, Limburg et al. analyzed data from the National Longitudinal Study of Adolescent to Adult Health and found that sexual and gender minorities have increased disparities in preconception care with increased unmet medical needs [22]. Stroumsa in an editorial in the Journal of Women's Health describes how discrimination leads to increased minority stress, which may be a cause of preconception care disparities [23]. Addressing these issues can directly improve the health of the patient and their potential future infant; it can also improve patient experience, engagement in care, and long-term patient–provider interactions.

Standard preconception begins with screening for potential future pregnancy in routine health maintenance visits. Transmasculine individuals with pregnancy potential should be asked at every visit if they plan on getting pregnant in the next year. Those who screen positively should get standard preconception counseling offered to cisgender people. The goal of prepregnancy care is to identify and reduce the risk of health effects on the person, fetus, and neonate. Aspects of prepregnancy counseling should include screening for chronic disease that can lead to high risk pregnancy, ensuring up-to-date immunization status, STI screening, substance and alcohol use screening, screening for housing and food insecurity, nutritional and BMI status. Patients should also be offered genetic screening pertaining to their ethnicity and universally for cystic fibrosis and spinal muscular atrophy [24, 25]. Prepregnancy counseling unique to transmasculine people includes gender-affirming hormone use, use of non-gendered language, and awareness around minority stress and trauma-informed care.

Testosterone

The National Transgender Discrimination Survey, a 70-question survey of 7500 transgender people, found that 69% of transgender men accessed hormonal care for gender affirmation [15]. When initiating testosterone, clinicians should counsel their patients that testosterone should not be considered a contraceptive. While there is no direct data on the effectiveness of testosterone in the prevention of pregnancy, there is some data to suggest that testosterone might be ineffective in preventing pregnancy. One qualitative study of 41 transmasculine people found that 5 became pregnant while still amenorrheic from testosterone [26]. A study on pregnancy intentions and outcome surveyed 1694 TGNB people and found that out of the 433 pregnancies in transmasculine individuals, 4 occurred while on testosterone [5].

Transmasculine people who desire pregnancy should be reassured that testosterone has not been shown clinically to affect ovarian reserve and that ovarian reserve markers remain within normal range while on testosterone therapy [27, 28] (see further detail in Chap. 3). However, testosterone has been designated a Class X teratogen by the FDA and has been associated with fetal anomalies in animal studies. Pregnant rats, exposed to testosterone, demonstrated offspring with hyperinsulinemia and skeletal muscle dysfunction [29]. In human studies, the only known effect is the virilization of 46XX fetuses, including labial fusion and clitoral enlargement. Data from gestational hyperandrogenism indicates that high levels of testosterone, such as in patients with luteomas, cause labial fusion and clitoral hypertrophy without other associated abnormalities [30]. There is no data on teratogenicity unrelated to genital anomalies in human studies.

Given this data, transmasculine people desiring pregnancy should be counseled to discontinue testosterone prior to and during pregnancy. While the pharmacokinetics of testosterone is well established, no data exists on the ideal washout period prior to attempting to conceive. Light et al. found that in their study, 80% ($n = 20$) resumed menstruation within 6 months after stopping testosterone [26]. The World Anti-Doping Agency recommends an 8-week washout period for athletes using testosterone cypionate prior to retesting for athletes receiving testosterone for hypogonadism [31]. The timeline to decreased testosterone levels is correlated with dose and methods of administration. Cessation of testosterone treatment should be balanced against parental well-being. Qualitative studies looking at the experience of transmasculine people attempting pregnancy show that stopping testosterone can cause increased gender dysphoria [7, 26]. Gender dysphoria refers to a feeling of intense emotional discomfort secondary to a mismatch between one's gender identity and their physical characteristics. Given the needed balance of necessary hormonal treatment and decreasing risk of exposure to a teratogen, it is our recommendation that pregnancy can be attempted as soon as ovulation occurs or within 1 month of discontinuing testosterone if cessation of testosterone causes stress or dysphoria for the patient.

Achieving Pregnancy

Transmasculine patients can use sperm from a partner, known donor, or anonymous sperm donor. Patients on long-term testosterone should be counseled about changes to reproductive anatomy. Conception methods and the effects of testosterone on reproductive anatomy is covered in detail in chapter (*Add Chap. 5)* in this book.

Preconception Screening

Cancer and STI Screening

All transmasculine people attempting to conceive should undergo standard preconception testing and screening. That includes identifying any issues in their overall health. Because of increased stigma and discrimination, TGNB people have been known to avoid regular health maintenance exams [6]. Providers should do a comprehensive history and physical exam and address any gaps in health maintenance. Particular attention should be given to comprehensive STI and HIV screening as untreated infections can affect the patient's health, decrease fertility, and have negative effects on the pregnancy and on the neonate. Complications of untreated STIs in pregnancy include: preterm premature rupture of membranes (Adjusted Odds Ratio [aOR] 1.35), postpartum sepsis (aOR 8.05), venous thromboembolic events (OR 2.21), need for cesarean delivery (aOR 3.06), and overall increased maternal mortality (OR 21.52). Adverse neonatal outcomes include preterm birth (aOR: 1.57), fetal death (OR 1.43), and fetal growth restriction (aOR 1.36) [32].

There are no data on HIV positivity rates specifically in transmasculine people attempting to conceive, but we know that due to stigma and decreased healthcare access, TGNB people as a group are disproportionately affected by STIs and HIV [6]. Data on transmasculine people indicate that the rate of HIV positivity is 3.2% [33], which is significantly higher than the 0.5% estimated rate of HIV in cisgender men [34]. Differences between these populations in sexual and other risk behaviors, along with other structural factors, may account for some of this difference in HIV+ rates. Given the high rates of HIV among transgender women (especially Black transgender women), as well as among men who have sex with men, any transmasculine person who is sexually active with partners with penises is at increased risk of HIV. HIV+ people should be counseled to undergo treatment with the goal of reaching an undetectable viral load prior to conception. For patients who are pregnant and are newly diagnosed with HIV, the goal would be to initiate therapy and reduce viral load to as low as possible. Data shows that vertical transmission declines as viral load declines. For patients with a viral load <400 copies/ml, the transmission rate has been shown to be around 1% and continues to decrease as viral load further decreases [35]. For new diagnosis in treatment-naive patients, recommendations include testing for drug resistance and initiation of empiric antiretrovirals until susceptibilities result. NIH recommendation includes dual NRTI backbone with a third drug consisting of either integrase inhibitor or a protease inhibitor. Dual NRTI backbone found to be safe in pregnancy and includes abacavir/lamivudine, tenofovir disoproxil fumarate/emtricitabine, or tenofovir disoproxil fumarate plus lamivudine. The integrase inhibitor recommended is dolutegravir or raltegravir. Protease inhibitors recommended in pregnancy include atazanavir + ritonavir or darunavir + ritonavir [36]. Of note, some observational data suggest a small increase in NTD with patients on dolutegravir prior to conception (increased from 0.08% to 0.3%), but no documented association with patients already on dolutegravir [37, 38]. Conversely, an animal study in zebrafish found that the partial antagonism on the folate receptor by dolutegravir is overcome by higher dose folate suggesting a role for high-dose folate [39].

Pap Smears

Prenatal visits provide the opportunity to ensure that transmasculine patients are up to date on cancer screening, including cervical cancer screening. Guidelines from USPSTF recommend that anyone with a cervix undergo cervical cytology with reflex HPV testing starting at the age of 21 [40] and co-testing (pap smear and HPV testing) at age 30 and older. Transmasculine people who have a cervix should be screened using the same guidelines. An additional consideration for transmasculine individuals includes awareness around testosterone-induced vaginal atrophy that can both make the exam more painful and has a ten times higher likelihood of yielding inadequate cells [41]. For patients with significant vaginal atrophy, administration of vaginal estrogens for 1–2 weeks prior to the exam may decrease the atrophic symptoms if acceptable to the patient [41]. As with patients of all genders, providers should also ensure that they use a trauma-informed approach to pelvic exams. Pelvic exams can be particularly traumatic for transmasculine people due to multiple factors, including the high rates of TGNB people who are survivors of sexual assault or abuse [6]. However, this is not the case for all patients and providers should not assume patients are uncomfortable with their anatomy or pelvic exams based on their gender identity alone. SAMHSA outlines techniques for trauma-informed pelvic exams. Components of a trauma-informed pelvic exam include: establishing rapport prior to the exam, allowing for support people in the exam room, discussing the procedure with the patient beforehand, informing the patient about each step in the exam prior to the exam, and empowering the patient to know that they can stop the exam at any point [18].

Substance Use

As part of routine prenatal care, providers should screen all patients for substance use issues. Substance use in pregnancy is associated with worse perinatal outcomes [42] and transgender people are three times more likely to report illicit substance use [6] with gender-related minority stress being a risk factor. The increased stress faced by gender and sexual minorities has a detrimental effect on their mental health and subsequently may lead to increased substance use [43]. Stigma by healthcare is a known risk factor for substance use in transgender people. Reisner et al. analyzed data from the US National Transgender Discrimination Survey (NTDS)—a 70 question survey of 75,000 transgender people across the USA—and investigated if gender minority stress was associated with higher rates of substance use specifically in order to cope with mistreatment ("I drink or misuse drugs to cope with the mistreatment I face or faced as a transgender or gender-nonconforming person"). 27.6% of respondents reported substance use to help cope with stigma and refused care. They found that enacted stigma (stigma by providers) leads to delays in routine preventive care (anticipated stigma). Mistreatment carried a risk ratio of 1.73 for substance use to cope with mistreatment [44]. Similar to preconception counseling with cisgender patients, TGNB people should be screened for substance use and offered support with any identified substance use issues prior to attempting pregnancy. It is important to note that substance use should never be a barrier to receive preconception counseling and prenatal care.

Intimate Partner Violence

TGNB people are disproportionally affected by Intimate Partner Violence (IPV). A systemic review found rates of IPV to be 1.7 times higher in TGNB individuals compared to cisgender individuals and that transgender people are 2.2 more likely to experience physical IPV and 2.5 more likely to experience sexual IPV [45]. While no data exists on IPV rates specific to pregnancy in transmasculine people, we know that pregnancy, in general, is a risk factor for increased IPV and it is reasonable to extrapolate to the TGNB population as well [46]. IPV causes both direct injury from violence and long-term mental and physical damage in the survivors. IPV is associated with an increased risk of adverse neonatal outcomes including lower birth weight (OR: 2.11), preterm birth (OR: 1.91), and small for gestational age (OR: 1.37) along with increased maternal and neonatal mortality [47, 48]. ACOG, as well as the USPSTF, American Academy of Family Physicians, and many other organizations recommend screening for IPV at the initial prenatal visits and at least once each trimester [49, 50].

Housing and Food Security

TGNB people are disproportionally affected by housing insecurity. A fifth of transgender people experience homelessness in their lifetime [15]. Transgender youth are disproportionally affected by housing insecurity and somewhere between 20 and 40% of homeless youth identify as LGBT+ [15]. Housing insecurity has been associated with low birth weight and/or preterm birth (RR: 1.73), Neonatal Intensive Care Unit (NICU) stay (RR: 1.64), and extended hospitalization (RR: 1.66) [51]. Providers should screen transgender people for housing security and refer them to appropriate social services in their prenatal visits.

TGNB people are also more vulnerable to food insecurity due to social and workplace discrimination and stigma. A survey of 105 transgender people in the Southeastern United States found that 79% have experienced food insecurity [52]. The USTS survey found that 12% of respondents relied on governmental food assistance like food stamps (SNAP) or WIC [6]. Food insecurity during pregnancy has been associated with multiple pregnancy complications including severe pregravid obesity (aOR 2.97), gestational diabetes (OR 2.76), and low birth weight in neonates (OR 3.2) [53, 54]. Providers should screen TGNB people for food insecurity and refer them to appropriate social services and food banks.

Prenatal Vitamins

The risk for neural tube defects (NTDs), including spina bifida, meningocele, and meningomyelocele, can be decreased with folic acid supplementation. USPSTF recommends that all women of reproductive age should be taking a prenatal multivitamin daily with at least 400 mcg of folic acid [55]. Light et al.'s study of 41 pregnant transmasculine patients found that 15% were not taking prenatal multivitamins during the first trimester [26]. Folate dosing includes 0.4, 1, and 4 mg, stratified by low, moderate, and high risk of NTD, respectively. Low risk is anyone with pregnancy potential. Moderate risk (1 mg) includes a family history of NTD, Type 1 or 2 diabetes, anyone on valproic acid or carbamazepine. High risk (4 mg) is anyone with a personal history of NTD or a previous NTD pregnancy [56]. High-dose folic acid supplementation should not be taken through a multivitamin, as higher doses of lipid-soluble vitamins like Vitamin A can be harmful to the fetus. These recommendations should be extended to all people with a uterus, who have or may have sex with pregnancy potential.

BMI and Health Weight Gain

BMI prior to pregnancy and gestational weight gain (GWG) are associated with the health of the pregnant person and their infant. Recommendations from the Institute of Medicine are dependent on pre-pregnancy BMI. For people with a BMI <18.5, recommended GWG is 28–40 lbs, BMI 18.5–24.9, recommended GWG is 25–35 lbs, BMI between 25 and 29.9 recommended GWG is 15–25 lbs and BMI >30, recommended GWG is 11–20 lbs [57]. As noted above, TGNB people are disproportionally affected by food insecurity, which can lead to inadequate nutrition during pregnancy. Clinics should screen for food insecurity and provide resources to dieticians, governmental food assistance and/or local resources.

Summary Preconception care for transmasculine people who are at risk or desire to become pregnant should include standard prenatal screening with particular attention paid to the disparities transgender people might face in society. Unique considerations to address include deliverance of care in a non-gendered manner and pausing gender-affirming hormones.

Identity and Mental Health

Pregnancy and childbirth are a time of increased emotional stressors for anyone. Rates of depression and anxiety increase during pregnancy and are reported to affect up to 11.9% of pregnancies [58]. Rates of postpartum depression and anxiety are even higher, approaching 21.9% [59]. Pregnancy for TGNB individuals comes with additional unique challenges. Transmasculine people are required to stop gender-affirming hormones prior to and for the duration of their pregnancy. This has been found to be a source of dysphoria for some, since stopping testosterone is associated with regression of masculine features (reduced facial hair growth), and return of feminization (resumption of menses prior to pregnancy, increased chest tissue growth, and widening hips) [60]. Even those who have had chest masculinization surgery (i.e., bilateral mastectomy) might experience increased chest growth. In Macdonald et al.'s qualitative study, they found that out of the nine respondents who had chest masculinization, six reported increased chest growth during pregnancy, some even to pre-surgery size. Patients should also be counseled that chest binding might be more painful due to pregnancy-related changes [7, 60]. These changes may cause some TGNB people to experience dysphoria. Pregnancy can make it more difficult to be perceived as one's affirmed gender, leading to potential misgendering and enacted transphobia. Lastly, preconception and prenatal care (and for some people, fertility care) might require them to disclose that they are transmasculine to healthcare providers when they otherwise may choose not to. All these factors, individually or combined, may negatively affect mental health through decreased affirmation and increased stigma [61].

Disclosure

Every transmasculine pregnant patient should consider how they want to address disclosure through pregnancy. A meta-synthesis study looking at how transgender people experience pregnancy found that pregnant transmasculine people have a variety of approaches. Some choose to be open about their gender and their pregnancy, some choose to present as women while they are pregnant, and others choose to hide the pregnancy with clothing. Each of these approaches comes with unique challenges. Choosing to disclose the pregnancy and to continue to present masculine opens one up to increased stigma, transphobia, discrimination, and potentially violence once pregnancy is visible. Choosing to present feminine can increase gender dysphoria, and worsen mental health through decreased affirmation. Hiding the pregnancy can limit social support from family and friends, as well as the social capital reserved for pregnant women [62, 63]. This situation tends to be worse for pregnant BIPOC people and for pregnant people with lower socio-economic status [64]. Providers should address this in their initial prenatal and preconceptions visits by eliciting the patient's thoughts on how they plan on handling disclosing their pregnancy status and screen for safety and support around those decisions.

Antepartum Considerations

Pelvic Exams

Pelvic exams are a necessary component of medical care in pregnancy and especially in labor. As outlined above, pelvic exams can be a significant source of stress for transmasculine individuals. Providers should ensure that pelvic exams are only performed when necessary and when relevant clinical information to care for patients cannot be obtained in another manner. Providers should also be versed in trauma-informed pelvic exams and screen for trauma history prior to exams.

Pregnancy Outcomes

There is a paucity of data on outcomes of pregnancy among transmasculine people. However, there are several reasons to assume that transmasculine people may be at increased risk for pregnancy complications. Social determinants of health such as poverty, homelessness, and food insecurity are associated with increased risk for preterm labor and low birth weight [65]. Indirectly, stigma and minority stress are hypothesized to lead to increase in substance use as a coping mechanism which can have multiple negative effects on maternal and perinatal outcomes, including fetal growth restrictions, preterm labor, placental abruption, and hypertensive disorders of pregnancy [44, 65]. Lastly, a large body of evidence points to minority stress as causative of worse obstetric outcomes, through allostatic load and neuroendocrine pathways [66]. Gender minority stress may likely have similar effects. All these risks are compounded by intersecting identities and therefore likely to differentially affect BIPOC TGNB people. Given the major disparities in maternal morbidity and mortality by race and ethnicity, BIPOC transmasculine people are likely to have higher rates of obstetric complications than their white cisgender peers.

While additional data are needed, there are a few studies that do look at pregnancy outcomes and complications in transmasculine people. In a study, Moseson et al. administered a cross-sectional self-administered survey and investigated the outcomes of 433 pregnancies in TGNB people. They found that 39% ended in a live birth, 33% in miscarriage, and 21% in abortion [5]. In another small study ($n = 41$), Light et al. looked at pregnancy complications rates in transmasculine people. Rates of complications differed from those in the general population, including: hypertension (12 vs. 2–8%) [67], preterm labor (10 vs. 12%) [68], anemia (7 vs. 16.16) [26, 69], and placental abruption (10 vs. 1–3.8%) [70]. Of note, this is a small non-representative, non-controlled sample in a qualitative study. Conclusions cannot be drawn as to prevalence of any of these complications in this population. Of note, none of the participants who were on testosterone prior to conceiving experienced anemia, most likely due to the effect of testosterone on hematopoiesis. That same study found that pregnancy, delivery, and birth outcomes did not differ between those who had used testosterone and those that didn't. Additional research is urgently needed to investigate pregnancy outcomes among TGNB people. Population-based, insurance claims-based, or multicenter studies may offer opportunities to assess the risks of obstetric complications and enable tailoring of preconception and prenatal care to the specific needs of transmasculine people.

Since access to reproductive services and supportive social networks are limited for many TGNB people, it is also possible that among the population of transmasculine people carrying pregnancies many of these risk factors are less prominent, and that this population is not representative of the general transmasculine population. Additional studies are needed to identify the unique needs of transmasculine individuals who conceive.

Delivery

Location of Delivery

Most deliveries in the USA occur within the hospital and with physician providers, with 9.8% choosing to deliver with a midwife and 1% delivering at home [71]. Based on a single cross-sectional qualitative study of 41 transmasculine people who had been pregnant and delivered a neonate, it appears that transmasculine pregnant patients have higher rates of both home births and delivery with a midwife. That study found that 17% of transmasculine pregnant patients choose to deliver at home, 28% delivered with a certified nurse-midwife, and 18% with a lay midwife [26]. That study also found that their choice of healthcare provider was motivated by the provider's acceptance of the person's identity. These findings support addressing transphobia, gender affirmation, and knowledge of TGNB pregnancy among a broad variety of practitioners who provide obstetric care.

Mode of Delivery

Indications for mode of delivery do not differ between TGNB and cisgender people. However, it is possible that a greater proportion of transmasculine people will choose to undergo an elective cesarean delivery. In a survey of 41 pregnant transgender people, 14.6% reported that they underwent an elective cesarean delivery [26]. This is compared with estimated rates at 2.5% in the USA [72]. Reasons for elective cesarean by request might be related to being uncomfortable with their genitals being examined and exposed and due to fear of increased dysphoria related to vaginal delivery. Overall in the study, rates of cesarean delivery vs. vaginal delivery were similar to those of the general US population, with 30% of deliveries occurring via cesarean delivery. Of the C-sections performed, 25% ($n = 3$) were requested by the patient [26]. When a patient expresses a preference for a cesarean delivery, providers should inquire about the motivation and counsel appropriately. In the absence of parental or fetal indication for C-section, vaginal delivery should be recommended. But ultimately, the patient's preference should be honored. For patients who elect to deliver via cesarean delivery, they should be counseled on the risks of repeat cesarean including placenta accreta spectrum disorder requiring cesarean hysterectomy, as these risks increase with each subsequent cesarean delivery [72].

Analgesia

All pregnant people must be counseled on pain control options during childbirth. Because of how fear of childbirth is heightened by gender minority stress, pain around childbirth can increase that fear. One qualitative study ($n = 17$) found that most respondents reported that the fear of pain was a central component of most participants' fear of childbirth [12]. Patients should be counseled on the various pain control options during their prenatal visits. Pharmacologic options include systemic and locoregional analgesia. Regional options include neuraxial analgesia and/or a pudendal nerve block. Systemic options include opioid analgesia, which is associated with greater side effects in both the laboring person and the fetus. Inhaled nitrous oxide can also be offered either as a primary or supplementary form of pain control. Non-pharmacologic pain management options include mindfulness, water immersion, Transcutaneous Electrical Nerve stimulation (TENS), movement and position changes and counter-pressure [73].

Providers should ensure that all their patients are offered comprehensive counseling about analgesia options and are given the opportunity to have their concerns about the pain of childbirth addressed. Providers should also emphasize that childbirth is unpredictable and that if their preferences change at any point they should feel empowered to advocate for optimal pain control.

Support

Pregnancy for transmasculine people can be an intensely isolating and lonely experience. A qualitative study ($n = 8$) found that feelings of loneliness were present in all of their respondents [7]. Social views of pregnancy as a feminine process and experience and the absence of visibility of pregnant transgender people might contribute to this isolation, which can be further exacerbated by lack of social support. Providers can help by creating a gender-neutral prenatal and birth space and connecting their patients with online and local support groups. Gender minority stress also plays a role in exacerbating fear around childbirth. Malmquist et al. explored how norms around maternity and femininity add an additional layer of stress to the fear of childbirth in LBT people. Hoffkling, in his qualitative study on how transgender men experience pregnancy ($n = 10$), writes how many of the respondents relied on community support groups to navigate their pregnancies. Several mentioned how helpful they found social media groups such as *Birth and Breastfeeding trans people and allies*, both during pregnancy and the postpartum period [63].

In summary, antepartum care of transmasculine patients is similar to that of their cisgender counterparts. To improve their experiences, clinicians should work to create more inclusive clinics and birth centers to reduce the associated discrimination. Additional data are needed to assess the outcomes of pregnancies in transmasculine people.

Postpartum

Lactation

Prior to addressing lactation with TGNB patients, providers should enquire about appropriate terminology regarding their chest anatomy. Macdonald et al. found that 91% (20/22) of transmasculine people surveyed used the term chestfeeding [60].

One unique concern with chestfeeding is the possibility that it can cause increased dysphoria. One qualitative study, which interviewed 6 transmasculine individuals, found that breasts tend to be the biggest source of gender dysphoria [74]. In Macdonald's study, 16 people attempted to chest feed, 7 experienced increased dysphoria, including 2 that stopped chestfeeding due to severe dysphoria. 9/16 reported no increase in dysphoria.

For transmasculine people who underwent chest masculinization surgery, there are additional considerations for lactation. The USTS found that 36% of transgender men undergo chest masculinization as part of their gender-affirming care, and 61% would want it 1 day [6], though the rates might be lower among transgender people carrying a pregnancy. The ability to lactate after chest surgery will depend on the surgical method. Surgeries with nipple grafting disconnect the nipple stalk and chestfeeding will not be possible. For those who have nipple-sparing procedures, lactation can be attempted.

For transmasculine patients who are unable to chest feed using their own anatomy, they can consider using supplemental nursing systems that allow one to simulate chestfeeding with either donor human milk or formula.

As with cisgender lactation, transmasculine patients should be counseled that inability to chest feed should not be considered a failure. While the benefits of lactation have been well documented, it can be a source of great stress, which can impact the mental health of the new parent during an already stressful postpartum period. Donor milk banks can also be considered so that the infant can receive the physiological benefits of human milk. If the child is co-parented with a person who has breasts, there are several protocols for induction of lactation among non-pregnant people with breasts (including cisgender women, transfeminine people, and transmasculine).

Induction of Lactation in Transfeminine People

Transfeminine people might not think that chestfeeding is possible because of the mistaken assumption that only people who were assigned female at birth can lactate. There are case reports of both cisgender women and transfeminine people inducing lactation to care for a neonate they adopted or carried by a partner or surrogate. The process involves months of increasing doses of estradiol, progesterone, and domperidone, along with nipple stimulation using a breast pump [75]. The latter drug is not available in the USA, is associated with risk of cardiac arrythmias, and may not impart the desired effect. Transfeminine people can safely continue using their gender-affirming hormones while chest feeding. Spironolactone is considered safe in lactation and is only minimally secreted in human milk [76].

Restarting GAH

Transmasculine people can restart gender-affirming hormones immediately in the postpartum period. Testosterone can suppress lactation in a dose-dependent fashion, where lower doses can allow for milk production but higher doses will suppress lactation [77]. There are case reports where 2 women diagnosed with theca lutein cysts were able to lactate once their testosterone range fell below 300 ng/dl [78]. Glaser et al. reported a case where a woman was treated with low-dose testosterone for depression. The studies did find low levels of testosterone in breastmilk, but because of the low oral bioavailability of testosterone, infant levels remained undetected [79]. Further research is needed to investigate if transmasculine people can initiate or restart their gender-affirming hormones and still chest feed.

Transdermal androgens: Patients on transdermal androgen gels (AndroGel, etc.) should be cautioned to apply the gel to an area where their infant would not be exposed when held or chest fed.

Postpartum Depression

The postpartum period is a particularly difficult time for new parents. Physical changes after childbirth along with the psychosocial changes involved in becoming a new parent contribute to risk factors for developing postpartum depression (PPD). While there are no data on the prevalence of postpartum depression in the transmasculine population, we know that due to transphobia, stigma, and access issues, TGNB people have a greater risk for depression and anxiety [15]. Additionally, one randomized control study of 121 cisgender women found an association with higher serum levels of testosterone and positive postpartum depression screening via Edinburgh Postpartum Depression Screen [80]. For transmasculine people, this can translate to a higher risk of developing PPD. Providers should screen for PPD at every visit and inquire about protective factors like social support. Clinics should also provide gender-neutral PPD support and resources.

Contraception

As noted, testosterone alone should not be considered an adequate form of contraception. Transmasculine people who engage in sexual activity with pregnancy potential should be offered contraception. While all forms of contraception are considered safe and efficacious in transgender men, there are some psychosocial considerations that can impact contraceptive choice. Estrogen and/or progesterone-containing pills and devices might be perceived as female hormones. Intrauterine devices require pelvic exams and procedures that can be a significant cause of distress, though certainly not universally [81]. Patients should be asked about their contraception plan prior to childbirth and during their postpartum visits. Contraception counseling should involve shared decision-making where the patient's values and preferences are elicited and all contraception options are presented for the patient to make a fully informed individualized contraception plan [82].

Summary

As we gain more information about the experiences of pregnancy care for TGNB people, more research is needed to identify and address the unique needs of this population. As academic institutions gather more data on this unique population, the findings confirm the narratives about how transmasculine people navigate pregnancy and/or healthcare. The majority of pregnancy care of transmasculine people follows the same principles of prenatal, preconception, antepartum, and postpartum care afforded to their cisgender counterparts. Unique needs of pregnant transmasculine individuals include accounting for body dysphoria during their care, chestfeeding, and gender-affirming hormones.

Providers and staff can improve their care by ensuring that practices are inclusive of all identities, practice trauma-informed care, and account for how racial and gender minority stress impacts the health of minorities. Awareness and addressing the barriers that TGNB people face in society and in healthcare can allow us to improve the care and health of our TGNB patients.

References

1. Sharman Z, editor. The remedy: queer and trans voices on health and health care. 1st ed. Vancouver: Arsenal Pulp Press; 2016. 256 p
2. Schneider DM. American kinship: a cultural account. Chicago: University of Chicago Press; 1980. 149 p
3. Weston K. Families we choose: lesbians, gays, kinship. New York: Columbia University Press; 1997 [cited 2020 Dec 30]. Available from http://ebookcentral.proquest.com/lib/umichigan/detail.action?docID=991398
4. Jackson Levin N, Kattari SK, Piellusch EK, Watson E. "We just take care of each other": navigating 'chosen family' in the context of health, illness, and the mutual provision of care amongst queer and transgender young adults. Int J Environ Res Public Health. 2020;17(19):7346.
5. Moseson H, Fix L, Hastings J, Stoeffler A, Lunn MR, Flentje A, et al. Pregnancy intentions and outcomes among transgender, nonbinary, and gender-expansive people assigned female or intersex at birth in the United States: results from a national, quantitative survey. Int J Transgend Health. 2020;22(1–2):1–12.
6. USTS-Full-Report-FINAL.pdf [cited 2020 Dec 22]. Available from https://www.transequality.org/sites/default/files/docs/USTS-Full-Report-FINAL.PDF

7. Ellis SA, Wojnar DM, Pettinato M. Conception, pregnancy, and birth experiences of male and gender variant gestational parents: it's how we could have a family. J Midwifery Womens Health. 2015;60(1):62–9.
8. Stroumsa D, Wu JP. Welcoming transgender and nonbinary patients: expanding the language of "women's health". Am J Obstet Gynecol. 2018;219(6):585.e1–5.
9. Singer RB, Crane B, Lemay EP, Omary S. Improving the knowledge, attitudes, and behavioral intentions of perinatal care providers toward childbearing individuals identifying as LGBTQ: a quasi-experimental study. J Contin Educ Nurs. 2019;50(7):303–12.
10. Tan KKH, Treharne GJ, Ellis SJ, Schmidt JM, Veale JF. Gender minority stress: a critical review. J Homosex. 2020;67(10):1471–89.
11. Christian R, Mellies AA, Bui AG, Lee R, Kattari L, Gray C. Measuring the health of an invisible population: lessons from the Colorado transgender health survey. J Gen Intern Med. 2018;33(10):1654–60.
12. Malmquist A, Jonsson L, Wikström J, Nieminen K. Minority stress adds an additional layer to fear of childbirth in lesbian and bisexual women, and transgender people. Midwifery. 2019;79:102551.
13. Stroumsa D, Roberts EFS, Kinnear H, Harris LH. The power and limits of classification—a 32-year-old man with abdominal pain. N Engl J Med. 2019;380(20):1885–8.
14. Rosenthal L, Lobel M. Explaining racial disparities in adverse birth outcomes: unique sources of stress for Black American women. Soc Sci Med. 2011;72(6):977–83.
15. Grant JM, Motter LA, Tanis J. Injustice at every turn: a report of the national transgender discrimination survey. 2011 [cited 2020 Dec 11]; Available from https://dataspace.princeton.edu/handle/88435/dsp014j03d232p
16. Craig SL, Austin A, Levenson J, Leung VWY, Eaton AD, D'Souza SA. Frequencies and patterns of adverse childhood events in LGBTQ+ youth. Child Abuse Negl. 2020;107:104623.
17. Felitti VJ, Anda RF, Nordenberg D, Williamson DF, Spitz AM, Edwards V, et al. Relationship of childhood abuse and household dysfunction to many of the leading causes of death in adults: the Adverse Childhood Experiences (ACE) study. Am J Prev Med. 1998;14(4):245–58.
18. SAMHSA's concept of trauma and guidance for a trauma-informed approach:27. 2014.
19. Guttmacher Institute. Abortion incidence and service availability in the United States, 2017. 2019 [cited 2021 Jan 19]. Available from https://www.guttmacher.org/report/abortion-incidence-service-availability-us-2017
20. Jones RK, Witwer E, Jerman J. Transgender abortion patients and the provision of transgender-specific care at non-hospital facilities that provide abortions. Contracept X. 2020;2:100019.
21. Moseson H. Abortion experiences and preferences of transgender, nonbinary, and gender-expansive people in the United States. Am J Obstet Gynecol. 2020 [cited 2020 Oct 9]; Available from http://www.sciencedirect.com/science/article/pii/S0002937820311261
22. Limburg A, Everett BG, Mollborn S, Kominiarek MA. Sexual orientation disparities in preconception health. J Women's Health. 2020;29(6):755–62.
23. Stroumsa D, Johnson TRB. Improving preconception health among sexual minority women. J Women's Health. 2020;29(6):745–7.
24. Prepregnancy Counseling [cited 2020 Dec 21]. Available from https://www.acog.org/en/Clinical/Clinical Guidance/Committee Opinion/Articles/2019/01/Prepregnancy Counseling
25. ACOG. Carrier screening for genetic conditions. [cited 2021 Mar 5]. Available from https://www.acog.org/clinical/clinical-guidance/committee-opinion/articles/2017/03/carrier-screening-for-genetic-conditions
26. Light AD, Obedin-Maliver J, Sevelius JM, Kerns JL. Transgender men who experienced pregnancy after female-to-male gender transitioning. Obstet Gynecol. 2014 Dec;124(6):1120–7.
27. Moravek MB, Kinnear HM, George J, Batchelor J, Shikanov A, Padmanabhan V, et al. Impact of exogenous testosterone on reproduction in transgender men. Endocrinology. 2020;161(3):bqaa014.
28. Caanen MR, Soleman RS, Kuijper EAM, Kreukels BPC, De Roo C, Tilleman K, et al. Antimüllerian hormone levels decrease in female-to-male transsexuals using testosterone as cross-sex therapy. Fertil Steril. 2015;103(5):1340–5.

29. Carrasco A, Recabarren MP, Rojas-García PP, Gutiérrez M, Morales K, Sir-Petermann T, et al. Prenatal testosterone exposure disrupts insulin secretion and promotes insulin resistance. Sci Rep. 2020;10(1):404.
30. Hakim C, Padmanabhan V, Vyas AK. Gestational hyperandrogenism in developmental programming. Endocrinology. 2016;158(2):199–212.
31. World Anti-Doping Agency. TUE physician guidelines- male hypogonadism. 2019. Available from https://www.wada-ama.org/sites/default/files/resources/files/tuec_malehypogonadism_version6.2.pdf
32. Arab K, Spence AR, Czuzoj-Shulman N, Abenhaim HA. Pregnancy outcomes in HIV-positive women: a retrospective cohort study. Arch Gynecol Obstet. 2017;295(3):599–606.
33. Becasen JS, Denard CL, Mullins MM, Higa DH, Sipe TA. Estimating the prevalence of HIV and sexual behaviors among the US transgender population: a systematic review and meta-analysis, 2006–2017. Am J Public Health. 2019;109(1):e1–8.
34. U.S. Statistics. U.S. Statistics, 2020. HIVgov 2020 [cited 2021 Jan 21]. Available from https://www.hiv.gov/hiv-basics/overview/data-and-trends/statistics
35. Mandelbrot L, Tubiana R, Le Chenadec J, Dollfus C, Faye A, Pannier E, et al. No perinatal HIV-1 transmission from women with effective antiretroviral therapy starting before conception. Clin Infect Dis. 2015;61(11):1715–25.
36. ClinicalInfo. Overview. Recommendations for use of antiretroviral drugs during pregnancy. Antepartum care. Perinatal. [cited 2021 Feb 19]. Available from https://clinicalinfo.hiv.gov/en/guidelines/perinatal/overview-2?view=full
37. Zash R, Holmes L, Diseko M, Jacobson DL, Brummel S, Mayondi G, et al. Neural-tube defects and antiretroviral treatment regimens in Botswana. N Engl J Med. 2019;381(9):827–40.
38. Zamek-Gliszczynski MJ, Zhang X, Mudunuru J, Du Y, Chen J-L, Taskar KS, et al. Clinical extrapolation of the effects of dolutegravir and other HIV integrase inhibitors on folate transport pathways. Drug Metab Dispos. 2019;47(8):890–8.
39. Cabrera RM, Souder JP, Steele JW, Yeo L, Tukeman G, Gorelick DA, et al. The antagonism of folate receptor by dolutegravir: developmental toxicity reduction by supplemental folic acid. AIDS. 2019;33(13):1967–76.
40. US Preventive Services Task Force, Curry SJ, Krist AH, Owens DK, Barry MJ, Caughey AB, et al. Screening for cervical cancer: US Preventive Services Task Force recommendation statement. JAMA. 2018;320(7):674.
41. Peitzmeier SM, Reisner SL, Harigopal P, Potter J. Female-to-male patients have high prevalence of unsatisfactory Paps compared to non-transgender females: implications for cervical cancer screening. J Gen Intern Med. 2014;29(5):778–84.
42. Forray A. Substance use during pregnancy. F1000Research. 2016 [cited 2021 Feb 9];5. Available from https://www.ncbi.nlm.nih.gov/pmc/articles/PMC4870985/
43. Parent MC, Arriaga AS, Gobble T, Wille L. Stress and substance use among sexual and gender minority individuals across the lifespan. Neurobiol Stress 2018 [cited 2021 Mar 5];10. Available from https://www.ncbi.nlm.nih.gov/pmc/articles/PMC6430403/
44. Reisner SL, Pardo ST, Gamarel KE, Hughto JMW, Pardee DJ, Keo-Meier CL. Substance use to cope with stigma in healthcare among U.S. female-to-male trans masculine adults. LGBT Health. 2015;2(4):324–32.
45. Peitzmeier SM, Malik M, Kattari SK, Marrow E, Stephenson R, Agénor M, et al. Intimate partner violence in transgender populations: systematic review and meta-analysis of prevalence and correlates. Am J Public Health. 2020;110(9):e1–14.
46. Gazmararian JA, Lazorick S, Spitz AM, Ballard TJ, Saltzman LE, Marks JS. Prevalence of violence against pregnant women. JAMA. 1996;275(24):1915–20.
47. Alhusen JL, Ray E, Sharps P, Bullock L. Intimate partner violence during pregnancy: maternal and neonatal outcomes. J Women's Health. 2015;24(1):100–6.
48. Donovan BM, Spracklen CN, Schweizer ML, Ryckman KK, Saftlas AF. Intimate partner violence during pregnancy and the risk for adverse infant outcomes: a systematic review and meta-analysis. BJOG Int J Obstet Gynaecol. 2016;123(8):1289–99.

49. Intimate Partner Violence [cited 2020 Dec 23]. Available from https://www.acog.org/en/Clinical/Clinical Guidance/Committee Opinion/Articles/2012/02/Intimate Partner Violence

50. Dicola D, Spaar E. Intimate partner violence. Am Fam Physician. 2016;94(8):646–51.

51. Leifheit KM, Schwartz GL, Pollack CE, Edin KJ, Black MM, Jennings JM, et al. Severe housing insecurity during pregnancy: association with adverse birth and infant outcomes. Int J Environ Res Public Health. 2020;17(22):8659.

52. Russomanno J, Jabson Tree JM. Food insecurity and food pantry use among transgender and gender non-conforming people in the Southeast United States. BMC Public Health. 2020;20(1):590.

53. Borders AEBM, Grobman WAM, Amsden LBM, Holl JLM. Chronic stress and low birth weight neonates in a low-income population of women. Obstet Gynecol. 2007;109:331–8.

54. Laraia BA, Siega-Riz AM, Gundersen C. Household food insecurity is associated with self-reported pregravid weight status, gestational weight gain, and pregnancy complications. J Am Diet Assoc. 2010;110(5):692–701.

55. US Preventive Services Task Force, Bibbins-Domingo K, Grossman DC, Curry SJ, Davidson KW, Epling JW, et al. Folic acid supplementation for the prevention of neural tube defects: US Preventive Services Task Force recommendation statement. JAMA. 2017;317(2):183.

56. Wilson RD, Wilson RD, Audibert F, Brock J-A, Carroll J, Cartier L, et al. Pre-conception folic acid and multivitamin supplementation for the primary and secondary prevention of neural tube defects and other folic acid-sensitive congenital anomalies. J Obstet Gynaecol Can. 2015;37(6):534–49.

57. Weight gain during pregnancy. Committee Opinion No. 548. American College of Obstetricians and Gynecologists. Obstet Gynecol. 2013;121:210–2.

58. Woody CA, Ferrari AJ, Siskind DJ, Whiteford HA, Harris MG. A systematic review and meta-regression of the prevalence and incidence of perinatal depression. J Affect Disord. 2017;219:86–92.

59. Wisner KL, Sit DKY, McShea MC, Rizzo DM, Zoretich RA, Hughes CL, et al. Onset timing, thoughts of self-harm, and diagnoses in postpartum women with screen-positive depression findings. JAMA Psychiatry. 2013;70(5):490.

60. MacDonald T, Noel-Weiss J, West D, Walks M, Biener M, Kibbe A, et al. Transmasculine individuals' experiences with lactation, chestfeeding, and gender identity: a qualitative study. BMC Pregnancy Childbirth. 2016;16(16):106.

61. Glynn TR, Gamarel KE, Kahler CW, Iwamoto M, Operario D, Nemoto T. The role of gender affirmation in psychological well-being among transgender women. Psychol Sex Orientat Gend Divers. 2016;3(3):336–44.

62. Besse M, Lampe NM, Mann ES. Experiences with achieving pregnancy and giving birth among transgender men: a narrative literature review. Yale J Biol Med. 2020;93(4):517–28.

63. Hoffkling A, Obedin-Maliver J, Sevelius J. From erasure to opportunity: a qualitative study of the experiences of transgender men around pregnancy and recommendations for providers. BMC Pregnancy Childbirth. 2017;17(Suppl 2):332.

64. Kritsotakis G, Vassilaki M, Melaki V, Georgiou V, Philalithis AE, Bitsios P, et al. Social capital in pregnancy and postpartum depressive symptoms: a prospective mother–child cohort study (the Rhea study). Int J Nurs Stud. 2013;50(1):63–72.

65. Amjad S, MacDonald I, Chambers T, Osornio-Vargas A, Chandra S, Voaklander D, et al. Social determinants of health and adverse maternal and birth outcomes in adolescent pregnancies: a systematic review and meta-analysis. Paediatr Perinat Epidemiol. 2019;33(1):88–99.

66. Rodriquez EJ, Kim EN, Sumner AE, Nápoles AM, Pérez-Stable EJ. Allostatic load: importance, markers, and score determination in minority and disparity populations. J Urban Health. 2019;96(Suppl 1):3–11.

67. Gestational hypertension and preeclampsia [cited 2021 Jan 19]. Available from https://www.acog.org/en/Clinical/Clinical Guidance/Practice Bulletin/Articles/2020/06/Gestational Hypertension and Preeclampsia

68. Management of preterm labor [cited 2021 Jan 19]. Available from https://www.acog.org/en/Clinical/Clinical Guidance/Practice Bulletin/Articles/2016/10/Management of Preterm Labor
69. Prevalence of anaemia in pregnant women (%) [cited 2021 Jan 19]. Available from http://www.who.int/data/gho/data/indicators/indicator-details/GHO/prevalence-of-anaemia-in-pregnant-women-(-)
70. Oyelese Y, Ananth CV. Placental abruption. Obstet Gynecol. 2006 Oct;108(4):1005–16.
71. Martin JA, et al. Births: final data for 2018. Natl Vital Stat Rep. 2019;68(13):47.
72. Cesarean delivery on maternal request [cited 2020 Dec 28]. Available from https://www.acog.org/en/Clinical/Clinical Guidance/Committee Opinion/Articles/2019/01/Cesarean Delivery on Maternal Request
73. Czech I, Fuchs P, Fuchs A, Lorek M, Tobolska-Lorek D, Drosdzol-Cop A, et al. Pharmacological and non-pharmacological methods of labour pain relief—establishment of effectiveness and comparison. Int J Environ Res Public Health 2018 [cited 2021 Jan 11];15(12). Available from https://www.ncbi.nlm.nih.gov/pmc/articles/PMC6313325/
74. Dutton L, Koenig K, Fennie K. Gynecologic care of the female-to-male transgender man. J Midwifery Womens Health. 2008;53(4):331–7.
75. Reisman T, Goldstein Z. Case report: induced lactation in a transgender woman. Transgender Health. 2018;3(1):24–6.
76. Spironolactone. In: Drugs and lactation database (LactMed). Bethesda, MD: National Library of Medicine (US); 2006 [cited 2020 Dec 13]. Available from http://www.ncbi.nlm.nih.gov/books/NBK501101/
77. Testosterone. In: Drugs and lactation database (LactMed). Bethesda, MD: National Library of Medicine (US); 2006 [cited 2020 Dec 13]. Available from http://www.ncbi.nlm.nih.gov/books/NBK501721/
78. Hoover KL, Barbalinardo LH, Platia MP. Delayed lactogenesis II secondary to gestational ovarian theca lutein cysts in two normal singleton pregnancies. J Hum Lact. 2002;18(3):264–8.
79. Glaser RL, Newman M, Parsons M, Zava D, Glaser-Garbrick D. Safety of maternal testosterone therapy during breast feeding. Int J Pharm Compd. 2009;13(4):314–7.
80. Aswathi A, Rajendiren S, Nimesh A, Philip RR, Kattimani S, Jayalakshmi D, et al. High serum testosterone levels during postpartum period are associated with postpartum depression. Asian J Psychiatry. 2015;17:85–8.
81. Boudreau D, Mukerjee R. Contraception care for transmasculine individuals on testosterone therapy. J Midwifery Womens Health. 2019;64(4):395–402.
82. Dehlendorf C, Grumbach K, Schmittdiel JA, Steinauer J. Shared decision making in contraceptive counseling. Contraception. 2017;95(5):452–5.

Chapter 7
Fertility Preservation in Transgender and Non-binary Youth

Rebecca M. Harris, Michelle Bayefsky, Gwendolyn P. Quinn, and Leena Nahata

Introduction

Reproduction is considered a basic human right, and parenthood is a major life goal for many young adults [1]. Research shows infertility can impede psychosexual development and cause psychosocial distress [2, 3]. While most studies to date have been conducted in oncology, these findings can inform practice for TGNB diverse youth seeking medical and surgical interventions that may cause transient or permanent infertility.

TGNB youth may initially seek treatment with a gonadotropin releasing hormone agonist (GnRHa) in early puberty, to prevent development of unwanted secondary sex characteristics. These agents do not cause permanent effects on fertility but they do prevent maturation of gametes. In later stages of puberty, gender affirming hormones (GAHs), including testosterone and estrogen, are often used to induce masculinizing and feminizing effects, respectively. Concerns have been raised about fertility impairment after testosterone exposure, though several cases have recently been published of pregnancies during or after testosterone therapy [4]. Decreases in

---

R. M. Harris
Division of Endocrinology, Department of Pediatrics, Boston Children's Hospital, Boston, MA, USA
e-mail: rebecca.harris@childrens.harvard.edu

M. Bayefsky · G. P. Quinn
Department of Obstetrics and Gynecology, Grossman School of Medicine, New York University, New York, NY, USA
e-mail: michelle.bayefsky@nyulangone.org; Gwendolyn.quinn@nyulangone.org

L. Nahata (✉)
Division of Endocrinology, Department of Pediatrics, Nationwide Children's Hospital, The Ohio State University College of Medicine, Columbus, OH, USA
e-mail: Leena.nahata@nationwidechildrens.org

© The Author(s), under exclusive license to Springer Nature Switzerland AG 2023
M. B. Moravek, G. de Haan (eds.), *Reproduction in Transgender and Nonbinary Individuals*, https://doi.org/10.1007/978-3-031-14933-7_7

testicular volume and impairment of spermatogenesis have been noted in transgender women treated with estrogen therapy [5, 6].

Recent guidelines state providers should educate TGNB individuals about the potential infertility risks and fertility preservation options prior to initiating medical or surgical gender affirming treatments [7]. Fertility preservation options for youth include oocyte cryopreservation and sperm cryopreservation, with ovarian and tissue cryopreservation as the only options for pre-/early pubertal youth. The American Society for Reproductive Medicine recently lifted the experimental label from ovarian tissue cryopreservation, but few live births have been reported to date with tissue cryopreserved from pre-menarchal youth [8]. Testicular tissue cryopreservation remains experimental, as no human live births have been reported.

Research in TGNB adults shows many individuals desire genetic parenthood and are willing to pursue assisted reproductive technology [9–11]. In contrast, research conducted to date in TGNB youth shows lower rates of fertility preservation utilization [12]. Many TGNB adolescents report a preference for adoption and/or lack of desire to have children in the future [12]. Fertility counseling is particularly complex in this population, for multiple reasons including: limited data exist regarding long-term effects of hormonal therapies on gonadal function; established fertility preservation options may not be available due to young age/pubertal stage; interventions may be costly with minimal to no insurance coverage; many adolescents lack capacity for future oriented thinking/planning; fertility preservation protocols and procedures may worsen dysphoria; and decision-makers (i.e., youth and parents) must be congruent about the process. Ethical and legal dilemmas may arise when an adolescent and their parents' fertility preservation perspectives conflict with one another, creating challenges for the healthcare team. A recent national study among providers of TGNB youth showed barriers to fertility counseling, inconsistent knowledge (particularly with regard to fertility preservation options), and a desire for more training in this area [13].

In this chapter we will: (1) review the literature on effects of gender affirming medical and surgical interventions on fertility; (2) outline fertility preservation options based on reproductive anatomy and pubertal stage; (3) discuss psychosocial considerations with regard to fertility preservation in TGNB youth; (4) address ethical and legal considerations; and 5) provide recommendations for clinical practice.

Medical Considerations

The medical management of gender transition is tailored to the individual. TGNB youth who are in the very early stages of puberty (Tanner 2 or 3) can decide, with the support of their parents, to start a GnRHa to block natal puberty. This can occur as early as 8–10 years of age and can continue until 13–14 years of age, at which time they may start GAHs. Additionally, some individuals receiving exogenous estrogen remain on GnRHa therapy to help suppress endogenous testosterone. For other TGNB individuals, the decision to pursue medical therapy for gender transition may occur later, toward the end, or even after, the completion of natal puberty [7]. It is important to distinguish between these two patient populations as their options for fertility preservation differ [14, 15]. For individuals whose natal puberty is "blocked" with a GnRHa, maturation of their gametes is halted. The concern is that when treatment with a GnRHa is followed by GAHs, the gametes never have a chance to fully mature [16]. One study from the Netherlands showed that one-third of transgender females on estrogen could not produce a semen sample due to early pubertal stage [17]. However, there has been a case report of oocyte preservation while on GnRHa [18]. For early pubertal youth, or youth who started on a GnRHa in early puberty, the main options for fertility preservation are ovarian or testicular tissue cryopreservation. In both of these instances, one or a portion of a gonad is removed and frozen for future reimplantation or *in vitro* gamete maturation. As discussed above, ovarian tissue cryopreservation is no longer experimental but has lower rates of oocyte maturation in pre-pubertal compared with post-pubertal individuals (25.3% vs. 38.0%, respectively) [19]. Further, the rate of live births in pre-pubertal ovarian tissue cryopreservation has yet to be established. Testicular tissue cryopreservation remains experimental; protocols are being investigated using animal models [20, 21].

For TGNB individuals who undergo most or all of their natal puberty, the likelihood of successfully using their gametes to conceive biological children is greater. One option is to preserve gametes (i.e., sperm banking or oocyte cryopreservation) before starting GAHs [20, 22]. For transmasculine individuals, the effects of testosterone on fertility are still being investigated, but thus far studies show that cortical follicle distribution in the ovaries of transgender individuals on testosterone for more than a year remain normal and there is no difference between oocyte yield or maturity in transgender men compared to cisgender women [10, 23]. Additionally, it is possible to stop testosterone and conceive naturally [4]. There have also been reports of unplanned pregnancies in individuals taking testosterone, and as such medical providers should counsel patients to use contraception [24]. For transgender women, sperm volume, concentration, and motility are lower in individuals who have used estrogen in the past compared with cisgender controls and are even lower in individuals currently using estrogen [5]. It may therefore be more challenging for transgender women to have biological children using their gametes compared to transgender men.

It should be mentioned that surgical management of gender transition is also tailored to the individual [7]. For patients who desire gonadectomy, the consent process should include a discussion about permanent sterilization, with options to cryopreserve oocytes prior to surgery and/or ovarian tissue during the surgery. For patients who choose to undergo hysterectomy, there should be a discussion about the inability to bear children in the future. Given that individuals can opt to have gonadectomy or hysterectomy or both, counseling should be tailored to each decision.

There are also several alternative options for family planning, including surrogacy, egg or sperm donation, and adoption. These are beyond the scope of this chapter but should be discussed with each patient as part of the consent process before starting medical or surgical treatment for gender transition. It is not sufficient to merely mention these options; the potential hurdles for each should be discussed as well (e.g., cost, accessibility, potential discrimination against transgender individuals, etc.) [25].

Finally, it is important to acknowledge that there remain many unknowns in fertility preservation for TGNB individuals. For TGNB youth specifically, the cohort is relatively young, with older individuals only now approaching reproductive age. Further research in this population is paramount. Many of these patients will remain on GAHs for decades and we do not yet know the long-term effects of GAHs on fertility. Further, knowledge about how long it takes for fertility to return after stopping GAHs remains elusive.

Psychosocial Considerations

Much of what is known about psychosocial issues in fertility preservation comes from the field of oncology. Adolescents and young adults with cancer have varying risk of impaired fertility or infertility depending on: age at cancer diagnosis, type and stage of cancer, surgery, chemotherapy and/or radiation treatment type and duration, as well as the possibility of existence of infertility from birth or prior to the cancer diagnosis. The American Society of Clinical Oncology, The American Academy of Pediatrics, and the American Society for Reproductive Medicine all recommend that patients of reproductive age be counseled about potential fertility risks and offered referrals to reproductive specialists for counseling prior to receiving any gonadotoxic treatment [26–28]. The evidence for these guidelines is rooted in the knowledge that the majority of adolescent and young adult patients with cancer wish to have a biological child in the future or siblings for their existing child/children. Further evidence suggests remorse and regret among patients who were not counseled about potential infertility or who did not make use of fertility preservation methods [29]. Among patients who did receive counsel but opted not to pursue fertility preservation there was less reported regret, and counseled patients were more satisfied than patients who did not receive or recall receiving fertility preservation counseling [30].

Less is known about remorse and regret related to fertility and decision-making among TGNB youth. Surveys of adult TGNB persons suggest desire for biological children [11, 31]. Some TGNB adults have completed their family building prior to beginning gender affirming care and others have taken steps to preserve fertility so as to leave options open for the future [32]. However, while there are increasing numbers of TGNB youth seeking gender affirming care, some evidence suggests reproductive health and fertility counseling may be unavailable or inadequate [33]. Recent surveys of medical and mental health providers involved in the care of TGNB youth showed gaps in fertility-related knowledge, counseling practices, and referrals [13, 34].

The World Professional Association of Transgender Health and The American Society for Reproductive Medicine have stated the same reproductive options and fertility preservation methods should be offered to individuals at risk for fertility loss regardless of gender identity [35, 36]. The majority of respondents in a recent large survey of the public also agreed clinicians should assist TGNB people to understand fertility preservation options for future biological children [37].

The literature is now growing with several published cases of older adult transgender men opting for oocyte cryopreservation and/or pregnancy [38–40]. In contrast, studies among TGNB youth are more variable—North American studies report fertility preservation rates of <5% [12, 41, 42], while sperm banking rates have been higher in other regions, potentially due to sociocultural considerations or lower cost or more comprehensive insurance coverage [17, 43]. Additional findings suggest some TGNB adolescents would prefer to adopt or have no desire to have children in the future [44]. However, in one recent study, many of the TGNB youth surveyed acknowledged the possibility their perspectives on parenthood may change with time [45]. If comparisons can be made to the oncology population, many adolescents and young adults may developmentally lack the ability for future forward thinking. As a result, missed opportunities based on a decision made at a younger age may serve as a source of regret later.

Another aspect of future parenthood and fertility preservation is intersectionality. Intersectionality refers to the multiple interacting identities of an individual, including factors such as gender, race, social class, ethnicity, and sexual orientation. These identities reflect structures that differentially impact an individual's healthcare experience [46]. For youth who identify with a religion or social class that does not favor assisted reproductive technologies or who cannot afford the costs of these services, there may be a lack of social support or resources for these decisions [47]. Further, youth whose sexual orientation is fluid, not yet established, or who have never been in a sexual or romantic relationship, thinking about parenthood in any form may be developmentally challenging or dysphoric [48].

In this context, an important aspect of fertility counseling for TGNB youth is the use of appropriate and relevant language. Medical terms such as sperm and oocytes may not be understood or may trigger dysphoria. For example, a person who identifies as a woman may disassociate with the concept of their bodies' ability to make sperm [49]. Using terminology suggested by the youth may improve understanding and facilitate decision-making.

As more TGNB youth are seeking hormonal interventions at earlier ages, discussions about fertility preservation are becoming more clinically and ethically complex, due to time constraints, developmental considerations, and family dynamics. Despite guidelines stating fertility preservation should be offered routinely, recent studies indicate only a minority of TGNB adolescents and young adults have these discussions with their healthcare teams [50], and that more counseling is desired [51]. Evidence-based strategies are needed to inform fertility counseling for this population to mitigate the potential distress and regret associated with fertility loss after treatment, which is well-documented in other adolescent and young adult populations (e.g., those with cancer). Specifically, since adolescents and young adults with cancer have improved psychosocial outcomes as a result of pre-treatment fertility counseling [30], standardized approaches to fertility counseling should be developed for TGNB youth as well.

Ethical and Legal Considerations

Fertility preservation in minors, including TGNB youth, raises a host of ethical and legal questions. First and foremost is the issue of autonomy: how should TGNB youth take part in the decision to undergo fertility preservation? The ethics literature on medical decision-making on behalf of children converges on the notion that below the age of 7, children lack capacity to participate in medical decision-making. At 7 years old or greater, some children may have capacity to provide assent, meaning that they give permission for the treatment to proceed. As children approach adolescence, all patients who are minors should generally be asked to provide assent [52].

In certain circumstances, the adolescent's views may be determinative—for example, when the medical treatment in question relates to sexually transmitted infections, contraceptive services, or prenatal care, most states permit adolescents to consent for these services themselves [53]. One could argue that fertility preservation is also related to sexual activity and childbearing, and the adolescent should therefore be the primary decision-maker. However, fertility preservation aims to allow patients undergoing gonadotoxic therapy to have children *in the future*. It does not involve treating an adolescent who has already assumed the more "mature" role of requiring treatment or prevention for sexually transmitted infections or pregnancy. Moreover, the main reason that adolescents do not need parental permission for sexual health-related treatments is to ensure that they are not deterred from seeking care. This calculus does not apply to fertility preservation, since there is no concern about repercussions for behavior perceived to be risky or irresponsible [54].

Minors may also become primary decision-makers if they are deemed mature enough to make a particular decision. In some states, there are specific criteria that the minor must fulfill to be considered sufficiently mature, including age [55]. In other states, such as New York, there is no formal process to declare a minor "mature," and a medical provider can simply decide that the minor is able to make a choice for themselves [56]. One can imagine a role for this category in fertility preservation, for example if an older adolescent seeks to pursue or decline treatment against the wishes of his or her parents. In general, when parents and children disagree, an adolescent's refusal to undergo treatment should carry more weight when the treatment involves high risk and relatively low benefit, such as low likelihood of success or minor significance of the medical issue at stake [57]. This is consistent with the ethical principle of non-maleficence, since overriding an adolescent's refusal for a treatment that is unlikely to be very beneficial may cause more harm than good. For fertility preservation, the relative burden of the treatment depends on

7 Fertility Preservation in Transgender and Non-binary Youth

the child's anatomy and pubertal stage and can range from producing a sperm sample to undergoing more invasive options such as ovarian tissue cryopreservation or oocyte freezing. Similarly, the benefit depends on whether the treatment is experimental (such as testicular tissue cryopreservation), and how important biological parenthood is to a given adolescent. However, children and adolescents may also be limited in their ability to estimate the importance of biological parenthood to their future selves, as their views might change, and it could be reasonable to assume that the benefit of preserving future fertility is great in order to maintain an open future [45].

Even when parents and children both hope to pursue fertility preservation, the costs of treatment can be prohibitive for many families, which is a major justice consideration. Only ten states in the USA have laws requiring private insurers to cover fertility preservation prior to treatments that will cause "iatrogenic infertility," and most of these laws were written with pediatric cancer patients in mind [58]. While the broad language used in legislation could apply to TGNB youth undergoing treatment for gender dysphoria, it is unclear how legislation will be implemented with respect to transgender patients [59]. In states where coverage for fertility preservation is not mandated, coverage decisions are left up to each private insurer, and TGNB youth may find themselves not qualifying for the same coverage afforded to cancer patients. For patients who are insured by Medicaid rather than private insurers, there are no states that require Medicaid coverage for fertility preservation [60]. Studies outside of the United States have shown higher rates of fertility preservation in TGNB youth and have discussed the potential association with lower out-of-pocket cost [43] and improved insurance coverage [17].

A final consideration for fertility preservation in TGNB youth is who controls the stored gametes. Standard protocol is for the gametes to remain in storage and for the minor to assume control upon reaching adulthood. The stored gametes cannot be used without the permission of the patient once they become an adult. If the patient does not survive until adulthood (a more common scenario with cancer treatment than treatment of gender dysphoria), the gametes are typically discarded [61]. In very rare circumstances, when the child has left clear written instructions that the gametes can be used posthumously, parents can assume control and pursue fertility treatments with the frozen gametes. This is an uncommon and ethically questionable situation; by far the more common scenario is that the young adult continues to store the gametes until they are ready to use, donate, or discard them [62].

Summary and Clinical Recommendations

In summary, medical and surgical interventions for TGNB youth may negatively affect fertility to varying degrees. Clinical practice guidelines outline the need to provide timely counseling about infertility risk and fertility preservation options, yet counseling approaches remain inconsistent. Many studies show TGNB adults desire biological children, yet research in TGNB youth shows a minority endorse this goal and few pursue fertility preservation. Several barriers exist to fertility counseling and preservation among TGNB youth, including: lack of data on long-term effects of hormonal interventions on fertility and health of offspring; limited established fertility preservation options for youth in early stages of puberty; developmental challenges in making future oriented decisions; potentially discordant perspectives of pediatric patients and their parents; and cost of fertility preservation interventions. Some insurance programs will cover fertility preservation considering it to be iatrogenic from the gender affirming care, while others do not. Advocacy efforts may include writing insurance appeal letters and/or investigating charity or financial assistance programs such as BabyQuest Foundation, familyequality.org, or gayparentstobe.com. More research is needed to inform optimal approaches to counseling, to prevent psychosocial distress and regret that has been seen in other patient populations. Based on the available evidence, we would recommend the following:

1. Prior to initiating medical/surgical interventions that may impact future fertility, providers of TGNB youth should:
   (a) provide counseling about potential infertility risk, including what is known and unknown.
   (b) offer referrals to discuss fertility preservation options, including what is established vs. experimental.
2. Consider a multidisciplinary team approach (including medical and mental health providers) to explore the youth's reproductive goals and facilitate fertility preservation decisions within the family.
3. Use clinical approaches in fertility counseling that are sensitive to TGNB youth, including inquiring about preferred terminology for anatomy and considering strategies to minimize dysphoria.
4. Consult with a local ethics committee in cases where youth and parents' fertility perspectives are discordant or uncertain.
5. Recognize that advocacy efforts may be needed to address systemic barriers such as costs.

References

1. United Nations Population Fund. Reproductive rights are human rights: a handbook for national human rights insitutions. 2014.
2. Armuand GM, Wettergren L, Rodriguez-Wallberg KA, Lampic C. Desire for children, difficulties achieving a pregnancy, and infertility distress 3 to 7 years after cancer diagnosis. Support Care Cancer. 2014;22(10):2805–12.
3. Lehmann V, Keim MC, Nahata L, Shultz EL, Klosky JL, Tuinman MA, et al. Fertility-related knowledge and reproductive goals in childhood cancer survivors: short communication. Hum Reprod. 2017;32(11):2250–3.
4. Light AD, Obedin-Maliver J, Sevelius JM, Kerns JL. Transgender men who experienced pregnancy after female-to-male gender transitioning. Obstet Gynecol. 2014;124(6):1120–7.

5. Adeleye AJ, Reid G, Kao CN, Mok-Lin E, Smith JF. Semen parameters among transgender women with a history of hormonal treatment. Urology. 2019;124:136–41. https://doi.org/10.1016/j.urology.2018.10.005.
6. Matoso A, Khandakar B, Yuan S, Wu T, Wang LJ, Lombardo KA, et al. Spectrum of findings in orchiectomy specimens of persons undergoing gender confirmation surgery. Hum Pathol. 2018;76:91–9.
7. Hembree WC, Cohen-Kettenis PT, Gooren L, Hannema SE, Meyer WJ, Murad MH, et al. Endocrine treatment of gender-dysphoric/gender-incongruent persons: an endocrine society clinical practice guideline. J Clin Endocrinol Metab. 2017;102(11):3869–903.
8. Nahata L, Woodruff TK, Quinn GP, Meacham LR, Chen D, Appiah LC, et al. Ovarian tissue cryopreservation as standard of care: what does this mean for pediatric populations? J Assist Reprod Genet. 2020;37(6):1323–6.
9. Auer MK, Fuss J, Nieder TO, Briken P, Biedermann SV, Stalla GK, et al. Desire to have children among transgender people in Germany: a cross-sectional multi-center study. J Sex Med. 2018;15(5):757–67. https://doi.org/10.1016/j.jsxm.2018.03.083.
10. Adeleye AJ, Cedars MI, Smith J, Mok-lin E. Ovarian stimulation for fertility preservation or family building in a cohort of transgender men. J Assist Reprod Genet. 2019;36(10):2155–61.
11. Wierckx K, Van Caenegem E, Pennings G, Elaut E, Dedecker D, Van De Peer F, et al. Reproductive wish in transsexual men. Hum Reprod. 2012;27(2):483–7.
12. Nahata L, Tishelman AC, Caltabellotta NM, Quinn GP. Low fertility preservation utilization among transgender youth. J Adolesc Health. 2017;61(1):40–4. https://doi.org/10.1016/j.jadohealth.2016.12.012.
13. Tishelman AC, Sutter ME, Chen D, Sampson A, Nahata L, Kolbuck VD, et al. Health care provider perceptions of fertility preservation barriers and challenges with transgender patients and families: qualitative responses to an international survey. J Assist Reprod Genet. 2019;36:579–88.
14. Neblett MF, Hipp HS. Fertility considerations in transgender persons. Endocrinol Metab Clin North Am. 2019;48(2):391–402. https://linkinghub.elsevier.com/retrieve/pii/S0889852919300088
15. De Roo C, Tilleman K, T'Sjoen G, De Sutter P. Fertility options in transgender people. Int Rev Psychiatry. 2016;28(1):112–9. http://www.tandfonline.com/action/journalInformation?journalCode=iirp20%0A. https://doi.org/10.3109/09540261.2015.1084275.
16. Harris RM, Tishelman AC, Quinn GP, Nahata L. Decision making and the long-term impact of puberty blockade in transgender children. Am J Bioeth. 2019;19(2):67–9.
17. Brik T, Vrouenraets LJJJ, Schagen SEE, Meissner A, de Vries MC, Hannema SE. Use of fertility preservation among a cohort of transgirls in the Netherlands. J Adolesc Health. 2019;64(5):589–93. https://doi.org/10.1016/j.jadohealth.2018.11.008.
18. Rothenberg SS, Witchel SF, Menke MN. Oocyte cryopreservation in a transgender male adolescent. N Engl J Med. 2019;380(9):886–7. Available from http://www.nejm.org/doi/10.1056/NEJMc1813275
19. Fouks Y, Hamilton E, Cohen Y, Hasson J, Kalma Y, Azem F. In-vitro maturation of oocytes recovered during cryopreservation of pre-pubertal girls undergoing fertility preservation. Reprod BioMed Online. 2020;41(5):869–73.
20. Goossens E, Jahnukainen K, Mitchell R, van Pelt A, Pennings G, Rives N, et al. Fertility preservation in boys: recent developments and new insights †. Hum Reprod Open. 2020;2020(3):hoaa016.
21. Jung SE, Ahn JS, Kim YH, Kim BJ, Won JH, Ryu BY. Effective cryopreservation protocol for preservation of male primate (*Macaca fascicularis*) prepubertal fertility. Reprod BioMed Online. 2020;41(6):1070–83.
22. Chen D, Bernardi LA, Pavone ME, Feinberg EC, Moravek MB. Oocyte cryopreservation among transmasculine youth: a case series. J Assist Reprod Genet. 2018;35(11):2057–61.
23. De Roo C, Lierman S, Tilleman K, Peynshaert K, Braeckmans K, Caanen M, et al. Ovarian tissue cryopreservation in female-to-male transgender people: insights into ovarian histology

and physiology after prolonged androgen treatment. Reprod Biomed Online. 2017 [cited 2018 May 5];34(6):557–66. https://doi.org/10.1016/j.rbmo.2017.03.008

24. Light A, Wang LF, Zeymo A, Gomez-Lobo V. Family planning and contraception use in transgender men. Contraception. 2018;98(4):266–9. https://doi.org/10.1016/j.contraception.2018.06.006.

25. Harris RM, Kolaitis IN, Frader JE. Ethical issues involving fertility preservation for transgender youth. J Assist Reprod Genet. 2020;37:2453–62.

26. Oktay K, Harvey BE, Partridge AH, Quinn GP, Reinecke J, Taylor HS, et al. Fertility preservation in patients with cancer: ASCO clinical practice guideline update. J Clin Oncol. 2018;36(19):1994–2001.

27. Nahata L, Quinn GP, Tishelman AC. Counseling in pediatric populations at risk for infertility and/or sexual function concerns. Pediatrics. 2018 [cited 2018 Aug 1];142(2). Available from www.aappublications.org/news

28. Committee E, Society A. Access to fertility services by transgender persons: an Ethics Committee opinion. Fertil Steril. 2015;104(5):1111–5. https://doi.org/10.1016/j.fertnstert.2015.08.021.

29. Jayasuriya S, Peate M, Allingham C, Li N, Gillam L, Zacharin M, et al. Satisfaction, disappointment and regret surrounding fertility preservation decisions in the paediatric and adolescent cancer population. J Assist Reprod Genet. 2019;36(9):1805–22.

30. Chan JL, Letourneau J, Salem W, Cil AP, Chan SW, Chen LM, et al. Regret around fertility choices is decreased with pre-treatment counseling in gynecologic cancer patients. J Cancer Surviv. 2017;11(1):58–63.

31. De Sutter P, Kira K, Verschoor A, Hotimsky A. The desire to have children and the preservation of fertility in transsexual women: a survey. Int J Transgenderism. 2002;6:1–12.

32. Vyas N, Douglas C, Mann CSWC, Weimer AK, Quinn MM. Access, barriers, and regret surrounding fertility preservation among transgender and gender diverse individuals. Fertil Steril. 2020;113(4):e26–7.

33. Amir H, Yaish I, Oren A, Groutz A, Greenman Y, Azem F. Fertility preservation rates among transgender women compared with transgender men receiving comprehensive fertility counselling. Reprod BioMed Online. 2020;41(3):546–54.

34. Chen D, Kolbuck VD, Sutter ME, Tishelman AC, Quinn GP, Nahata L. Knowledge, practice behaviors, and perceived barriers to fertility care among providers of transgender healthcare. J Adolesc Health. 2019;64(2):226–34. https://doi.org/10.1016/j.jadohealth.2018.08.025.

35. World Professional Association for Transgender Health. Standards of care for transsexual, transgender, and gender non-conforming people. 7th version. 2012.

36. ASRM. Access to fertility services by transgender persons: an ethics committee opinion. Fertil Steril. 2015;104(5):1111–5.

37. Goldman RH, Kaser DJ, Missmer SA, Farland LV, Ashby RK, Ginsburg ES. Fertility treatment for the transgender community: a public opinion study. J Assist Reprod Genet. 2017;34(11):1457–67.

38. Armuand G, Dhejne C, Olofsson JI, Rodriguez-Wallberg KA. Transgender men's experiences of fertility preservation: a qualitative study. Hum Reprod. 2017 [cited 2018 May 5];32(2):383–90. Available from https://watermark.silverchair.com/dew323.pdf?token=AQECAHi208BE4 9Ooan9kkhW_Ercy7Dm3ZL_9Cf3qfKAc485ysgAAAaQwggGgBgkqhkiG9w0BBwaggg GRMIIBjQIBADCCAYYGCSqGSIb3DQEHATAeBglghkgBZQMEAS4wEQQMnielyD Aqm-F8Dwo9AgEQgIIBV2Ox53b115DVD5mISP0uKG1p-APYkC2yqwksT0kKGs1MfhDt

39. Maxwell S, Noyes N, Keefe D, Berkeley AS, Goldman KN. pregnancy outcomes after fertility preservation in transgender men. Obstet Gynecol. 2017;129(6):1031–4.

40. Insogna IG, Ginsburg E, Srouji S. Fertility preservation for adolescent transgender male patients: a case series. J Adolesc Health. 2020;66(6):750–3.

41. Chen D, Simons L, Johnson EK, Lockart BA, Finlayson C. Fertility preservation for transgender adolescents. J Adolesc Health. 2017;61(1):120–3.

42. Chiniara LN, Viner C, Palmert M, Bonifacio H. Perspectives on fertility preservation and parenthood among transgender youth and their parents. Arch Dis Child. 2019;104(8):739–44. Available from http://adc.bmj.com/lookup/doi/10.1136/archdischild-2018-316080
43. Pang KC, Peri AJ, Chung HE, Telfer M, Elder CV, Grover S, et al. Rates of fertility preservation use among transgender adolescents. JAMA Pediatr. 2020;174(9):890–1.
44. Tornello SL, Bos H. Parenting intentions among transgender individuals. LGBT Health. 2017;4(2):115–20. Available from http://online.liebertpub.com/doi/10.1089/lgbt.2016.0153
45. Nahata L, Chen D, Quinn G, Travis M, Grannis C, Nelson E, et al. Reproductive attitudes and behaviors among transgender/nonbinary adolescents. J Adolesc Health. 2020;66(3):372–4.
46. Nixon L. The right to (trans) parent: a reproductive justice approach to reproductive rights, fertility, and family-building issues facing transgender people. William Mary J Race Gender Soc Justice. 2013;20:73–103.
47. von Doussa H, Power J, Riggs D. Imagining parenthood: the possibilities and experiences of parenthood among transgender people. Cult Health Sex. 2015;17(9):1119–31.
48. Holmberg M, Arver S, Dhejne C. Supporting sexuality and improving sexual function in transgender persons. Nat Rev Urol. 2019;16(2):121–39.
49. Riggs DW, Bartholomaeus C. Transgender young people's narratives of intimacy and sexual health: implications for sexuality education. Sex Educ. 2018;18(4):376–90.
50. Baram S, Myers SA, Yee S, Librach CL. Fertility preservation for transgender adolescents and young adults: a systematic review. Hum Reprod Update. 2019;25(6):694–716.
51. Quain KM, Kyweluk MA, Sajwani A, Gruschow S, Finlayson C, Gordon EJ, et al. Timing and delivery of fertility preservation information to transgender adolescents, young adults, and their parents. J Adolesc Health. 2020;18:S1054-139X(20)30398-0.
52. Katz AL, Webb SA. Informed consent in decision-making in pediatric practice. Pediatrics. 2016;138(2):e20161485. Available from http://pediatrics.aappublications.org/cgi/doi/10.1542/peds.2016-1485
53. Committee on Adolescent Health Care. Committee opinion no 699: adolescent pregnancy, contraception, and sexual activity. Obstet Gynecol. 2017;129(5):e142–9.
54. Guttmacher Institute. An overview of consent to reproductive health services by young people. State policies in brief 2020. Available from https://www.guttmacher.org/state-policy/explore/overview-minors-consent-law
55. Coleman DL, Rosoff PM. The legal authority of mature minors to consent to general medical treatment. Pediatrics. 2013;131(4):786–93.
56. Feierman J, Lieberman D, Schissel A, Diller R, Kim J, Chu Y. Teenagers, health care and the law. New York Civil Liberties Union. 2018.
57. Kohrman A, Clayton EW, Frader JE, Grodin MA, Moseley KL, Porter IH, et al. Informed consent, parental permission, and assent in pediatric practice. Pediatrics. 1995;95(2):314–7.
58. Resolve. Infertility coverage by state. 2020 [cited 2020 Oct 26]. Available from https://resolve.org/what-are-my-options/insurance-coverage/infertility-coverage-state/
59. Kyweluk MA, Reinecke J, Chen D. Fertility preservation legislation in the United States: potential implications for transgender individuals. LGBT Health. 2019;6(7):331–4. Available from https://www.liebertpub.com/doi/10.1089/lgbt.2019.0017
60. Kaiser Family Foundation. Coverage and use of fertility services in the US. 2020.
61. Klipstein S, Fallat ME, Savelli S, Katz AL, MacAuley RC, Mercurio MR, et al. Fertility preservation for pediatric and adolescent patients with cancer: medical and ethical considerations. Pediatrics. 2020;145(3):e20193994.
62. Affdal AO, Ravitsky V. Parents' posthumous use of daughter's ovarian tissue: ethical dimensions. Bioethics. 2019;33:82–90.

Chapter 8
Non-procreative Reproductive Issues and Sexual Function in Transmasculine Individuals

Frances Grimstad

Transmasculine patients may present to gynecologists for non-procreative concerns and care. Gynecologists should be familiar with how gender identity and gender affirmation therapies and surgeries can influence this. Non-procreative aspects of transmasculine gynecology involve the spectrum of gynecologic care and may include pelvic pain, contraception, gender-affirming hysterectomies, or uterine bleeding on testosterone. While a great deal of data in these areas has emerged in recent years to inform the gynecologic care of transmasculine patients, much is still unknown. This chapter reviews non-procreative gynecology areas for transmasculine individuals, the data surrounding them, and initial evaluation and management approaches.

Gynecologic History and Physical Considerations in the Transmasculine Patient

A history and physical should generally proceed as per cisgender female guidelines with a few considerations. Clinicians should take a trauma-informed approach [1]. This includes allowing patients to be in control of if and when they discuss their medical history. Patients should be asked about any chosen terminology for their anatomy, reproductive physiology, and sexual activity (e.g., bleeding instead of menstruation, front hole instead of vagina). The history should include any past

F. Grimstad (✉)
Division of Gynecology, Department of Surgery, Boston Children's Hospital, Boston, MA, USA

Department of Obstetrics, Gynecology, and Reproductive Biology, Harvard Medical School, Boston, MA, USA
e-mail: frances.grimstad@childrens.harvard.edu

© The Author(s), under exclusive license to Springer Nature Switzerland AG 2023
M. B. Moravek, G. de Haan (eds.), *Reproduction in Transgender and Nonbinary Individuals*, https://doi.org/10.1007/978-3-031-14933-7_8

gender-affirming medical or surgical therapies or any desires for them in the present or future. Transgender patients experience high rates of trauma and violence and should be screened for them during evaluation [2].

A gender-inclusive sexual history should include asking about the patient's gender identity, sexual orientation, and whether they have engaged in sexual activity. Patients should be asked about the anatomic parts they and their partner(s) use during sexual activity and whether the patient or their partner(s) can produce sperm or eggs. Patients should also be asked about their reproductive goals, including present or future desires for pregnancy and any desires for genetically related children. Neither sexual activity nor desire for gamete usage should be assumed based on gender identity. Patients who identify as transmasculine can have diverse sexual orientations and may use different parts of their anatomy (including native or neo genitalia) when engaging in sexual activity [3–5].

Not everyone seen by a gynecologist is born with, or presently has, the same anatomy [6]. Some people are born with differences in sexual development, such as those who identify as intersex. Others may undergo surgeries that change their reproductive tract (e.g., hysterectomy) or genitals (e.g., phalloplasty) [2]. Assumption of an anatomic binary can risk gaps in care due to missed anatomic or physiological considerations. Using an anatomic inventory (Table 8.1) ensures anatomy past and present is considered during the course of the patient's care.

A discussion of recommendations regarding the exam components should occur. Clear guidance should be provided to patients regarding the rationale for each aspect of the physical exam and evaluation. Shared decision-making should be used to determine the exam approach [1]. This can include the use of harm reduction methods (e.g., self-swabs for infections, delaying speculum exams, or utilizing an abdominal ultrasound as a screening for evaluation of pelvic masses instead of an internal exam), or offering a support person [7]. It is important to note that not all TGNB patients are going to have dysphoria or difficulty with a pelvic exam. Clinicians should investigate which part of the encounter may be difficult for the patient without assuming they are uncomfortable with the exam or their anatomy.

Table 8.1 Genital and reproductive anatomic inventory (this list is not inclusive of all genital and reproductive anatomy but provides the key aspects which may inform differential diagnosis)

Anatomy	Has presently	Surgically removed	Surgically created	Never had	Unsure/ Unknown
Cervix					
Clitoris					
Clitorophallus					
Ovaries					
Penis					
Prostate					
Scrotum					
Testes					
Uterus					
Vagina					
Vulva					

Changes in Genital and Reproductive Anatomy and Physiology on Testosterone

Changes to the Uterus on Testosterone

Under cisgender male androgen levels, the endometrial environment is relatively hypoestrogenic and with low to no progesterone exposure [8]. This is predominately likely due to the suppression of ovarian function [9].

Androgen receptors are present in the endometrium [10]. In cisgender females their expression fluctuates during the menstrual cycle (thought to be mediated in part by estrogen and progesterone) with activity highest in the proliferative phase (particularly in the glands) and lowest in the early secretory phase. There is also a lower expression in the myometrium. In a transmasculine person on testosterone, the androgen receptor patterns appeared inverted, with the highest expression in the myometrium and stroma and lowest in the epithelium [11]. How they directly influence endometrial regulation in transmasculine patients on testosterone is unclear.

The uterine size in a transmasculine person on testosterone is similar to those of reproductive age cisgender women [8]. The endometrium is generally thin (<4 mm) [8, 12]. A mixture of histology is seen with some patients having inactive endometrium (tubular glands with cuboidal epithelium, low nucleo-cytoplasmic ratio, and compact stroma), and others proliferative (glandular proliferation, stratified columnar epithelium, high nucleo-cytoplasmic ratio, and number of mitotic figures, and cystically dilated glands) [8, 10]. Proliferative endometrium does not decrease in frequency with more extended testosterone usage, higher BMI, or older age [8]. High rates of ovulatory suppression likely contribute to a low progesterone environment and the lack of secretory endometrium [9].

Typical benign uterine masses continue to be found in transmasculine persons on testosterone, including polyps, leiomyoma, and adenomyosis [8]. Persistent endometriosis has also been identified [13]. Endometrial hyperplasia without atypia does not appear to be increased in frequency in persons on testosterone, with rare cases seen in large cohorts. Only one cohort study has had a single case of focal adenocarcinoma [8].

Changes to the Ovaries on Testosterone

The ovaries in transmasculine persons on testosterone exhibit a diversity of pathology. Certain studies highlight a preponderance of multicystic or polycystic morphology. Other studies note large numbers of atretic follicles. Simple cysts, ovarian fibromas, and endometriomas have also all been documented in transmasculine persons on testosterone [14]. Increased thickness of the tunica albuginea and collagenous layer and stromal hyperplasia has been seen [15]. Present studies do not document an increased risk of malignant pathology in ovaries on testosterone;

however, case reports of malignancies do exist, suggesting the risk is not absent [14]. The ovarian volume is typically within the normal range for cisgender reproductive age females (7.6–10.9 cm³) [14]. In one study, an inverse correlation has been identified between duration of testosterone use and ovarian volume [14]. While ovarian atrophy is found in some patients, numerous studies have documented successful use of eggs for pregnancy following discontinuation of testosterone in transmasculine patients, suggesting the majority of ovaries are not irreversibly impaired [16, 17]. This data will be reviewed in greater detail in Chap. 3.

Changes to the Vulva and Vagina on Testosterone

The hypoestrogenic environment on systemic testosterone can lead to vulvovaginal atrophy in some individuals. Lower rates of lactobacillus are found in vaginas on testosterone, likely due to estrogen shift [18]. The clitorophallus (the erectile organ, which may be called the clitoris or penis by some patients) also enlarges on testosterone and can increase up to 2 cm from the original length [19].

Changes to the Urinary System on Testosterone

Early data suggest that testosterone may be associated with increased bladder capacity and post-void residual volume. However, it is unclear to what degree this is related to androgens versus lifestyle changes experienced by transmasculine people (e.g., holding urine due to bathroom safety concerns) [20]. No data presently shows increased rates of urinary pathology. However, vulvovaginal atrophy is known to contribute to urinary tract infection frequency [21].

Gynecologic Considerations in Gender-Affirming Genital and Reproductive Surgeries

Hysterectomies in Transmasculine Patients

In the 2015 US Transgender Survey, 71% of transmasculine persons wanted or had already had a hysterectomy [2]. Some may desire it for the same reasons as cisgender women (e.g., leiomyoma), while others may desire it for gender-specific reasons [22]. Gender-specific reasons may include dysphoria related to the uterus, or interest in additional genital affirmation surgery for which a hysterectomy is an initial step (e.g., some but not all metoidioplasty, or phalloplasty) [23]. While hysterectomies are desired by some, not all will want to undergo the procedure and it is not required for persons on testosterone [22].

8 Non-procreative Reproductive Issues and Sexual Function in Transmasculine...

Hysterectomies for gender affirmation are technically no different than for benign gynecologic conditions [24]. Most are done minimally invasively, and a risk-reducing bilateral salpingectomy is typically performed. As with the shifting trend away from default oophorectomies in benign hysterectomies in cisgender women of reproductive age, oophorectomies are not required in hysterectomies done for gender affirmation (including for those done in preparation for metoidioplasty or phalloplasty) [22]. The choice of oophorectomy is an individualized decision. As discussed in Sect. 8.2.2, the ovaries are relatively suppressed on testosterone, and there is no increased frequency of malignant pathology [14]. No guideline recommends ovarian removal to aid in virilization [25]. Reasons to retain ovaries include:

- The patient desires a source of backup sex steroids, should they discontinue testosterone for any reason (including loss of access or personal choice) [2].
- The patient wants the option to use their oocytes in the future in a gestational carrier [26].

Reasons to remove ovaries at the time of gender-affirming hysterectomy include:

- The patient experiences dysphoria around retained ovaries.
- The patient is over the age where ovaries would have been retained for reduction in morbidity and mortality in cisgender women at the time of benign hysterectomy (typically over the age of 45–54 years) [27].
- The patient has a personal or family history that would qualify for a prophylactic bilateral salpingo-oophorectomy in a cisgender female of the same age.
- The patient has a history of ovarian pathology which would qualify for an oophorectomy in a cisgender female of the same age (e.g., borderline serous cystadenoma).

Patients should be counseled that ovaries can always be removed later should they desire to retain them at the time of hysterectomy.

Metoidioplasty and Phalloplasty

The most common transmasculine genital gender-affirming surgeries are metoidioplasty and phalloplasty [28]. These can occur with or without urethral lengthening or scrotoplasty. Both procedures may be preceded by a hysterectomy and vaginectomy, but this is not required by all surgeons and is individualized based on patient goals and priorities. Metiodioplasties use the hormonally enlarged clitorophallus as a base to create a small neophallus. Patients can also undergo urethral elongation using vulvovaginal tissues along the ventral aspect [29]. Most metoidioplasties allow patients to stand to void. The phalloplasty utilizes the foundation of the metoidioplasty procedure and builds upon it by adding a shaped soft tissue flap with an additionally lengthened urethra to create a larger neophallus. The clitoral sensory nerves are mobilized, and ilioinguinal or iliohypogastric nerves can also be utilized for additional sensory input.

Patients may ask gynecologists for support in postoperative care and evaluating complications. All of these complications should be managed by the original surgeon or a trained urologist. The most commonly reported complications are urethral (strictures, fistulae, and diverticula) [30, 31]. Signs of these conditions may include hematuria, pain, voiding dysfunction, or incontinence. Granulation tissue and scarring can also occur in either procedure [32]. Some patients may undergo testicular implants with these procedures with or without scrotoplasty. Others who have undergone phalloplasty may have erectile rods placed for erectile capacity. These implants and devices can become infected, migrate, or erode [33, 34].

The neophallus donor tissue is still susceptible to infections and lesions from its donor site. Patients should be asked about the skin's original site when assessing for any infections or lesions, and they should be worked up and managed as they would be for the original location. See Sect. 8.6 for information on sexually transmitted infections (STI) in neogenitalia.

Chest Care in the Transmasculine Patient

Masculinizing chest surgery is the most common gender-affirming surgery sought by transmasculine patients [35]. It removes the glandular breast tissue and creates a masculinizing chest contour [36]. Most patients report high satisfaction [37]. Long-term concerns may include loss of nipple-areola sensation. Patients may also have concerns about their scars. These should be referred back to the original surgeon or another plastic surgeon specializing in chest reconstruction. Published case reports discuss post-reconstruction patients who have successfully lactated and chest fed following pregnancy [38]. However, the frequency of success of this following chest reconstruction has yet to be ascertained and is likely related to the type of reconstruction performed, use of free nipple grafts, and amount of remaining glandular tissue.

Chest reconstruction surgery is not the same as a double mastectomy done for malignancy purposes because not all glandular tissue is removed [23]. Any masses should be worked up per cisgender female guidelines. Transmasculine patients following chest reconstruction still carry a risk for cancer, although present data suggests it is less than cisgender women [39]. Regardless, breast cancer has been diagnosed both pre- and post-chest reconstruction, and present guidelines do not recommend any deviation from cisgender female guidelines regarding breast cancer screening [23]. Clinicians should engage in shared decision-making with patients using available evidence to guide discussions about approaches to screening [23]. Mammography may be difficult as it requires tissue for compression. Clinicians should consult a breast radiologist and engage in shared decision-making with their patients regarding any modifications in approach (e.g., ultrasound) [40].

Human Papillomavirus and Cervical Cancer Screening in Transmasculine Patients

All patients, regardless of genitalia, are susceptible to Human Papillomavirus (HPV)-related pathology and should be counseled up to age 45 years on HPV vaccination [41]. Few cervical cancer cases have been reported in transmasculine persons on testosterone, which may be influenced by the population's hysterectomy rate [2]. Despite this, all persons with a cervix require cervical cancer screening, and protocols are as per cisgender female guidelines. Testosterone does cause a decrease in cervical cellularity, which can lead to inadequate Pap tests [42]. A longer duration of testosterone use is associated with a higher risk of inadequate Pap tests. For those who require repeat cervical cytology due to inadequacy, vaginal estrogen can be trialed before the Pap to try to improve cellularity [43]. High-risk HPV DNA primary screening over 30 years has been endorsed by ACOG as an alternative approach to cytology. Some patients may need moderate sedation or deep sedation in an operating room for pap smears while others will tolerate an office exam without difficulty [44]. Due to the concerns addressed in Sect. 8.1 regarding challenges with pelvic exams for some individuals, it is important to consider harm reduction approaches. For example, research in transmasculine patients found high concordance between clinician-performed HPV DNA vaginal swabs and patient self-swabs, suggesting that self-swabs are a possible alternative for patients who cannot tolerate a clinician-performed pelvic exam-mediated swab and for whom sedation is not an option due to cost, patient preference, clinic or operating room availability [45].

Sexually Transmitted Infections in Transmasculine Patients

Sexually transmitted Infection (STI) risk is related to anatomy and behavior and not identity. As per Sect. 8.1, clinicians should ask about gender identity, sexual orientation, the patient, and partner's present anatomy. The Center for Disease Control guidelines on special populations recommend focusing on anatomy and orifice-specific approaches to STI screening [46]. No present evidence suggests neogenitalia are not susceptible to STIs. These should continue to be considered on the differential of those who are sexually active. Neo-urethras made with vaginal mucosa likely continue to have a susceptibility to STIs, along with continued susceptibility of the upstream native urethra and bladder. However, the neo-urethra in the neophallus is likely more resistant to these infections due to keratinized squamous epithelium. Urine STI testing has not been validated in persons with neogenitalia, but it is reasonable to begin with this orifice.

Contraception Counseling and Transmasculine Patients

Some transmasculine patients may be at risk of unintended pregnancy (have a uterus, ovaries, and engage in unprotected penile-vaginal sex with a partner capable of producing sperm) and have a need for contraception [47, 48]. Over half of the transmasculine population has reported utilizing contraception [49]. This includes transmasculine persons on, and not on, testosterone. Despite a high prevalence of amenorrhea and early data showing a high rate of ovulation suppression, testosterone is not approved for contraception purposes. It is also considered a teratogen in pregnancy due to the virilizing effects that can occur in a fetus [50]. There is no present evidence to suggest that any type of contraception (Table 8.2) is contraindicated with testosterone use. As such all methods should be offered to patients.

Clinicians should utilize the gender-affirming history (Sect. 8.1) to ascertain whether the patient is at risk for unintended pregnancy and to inform contraceptive counseling. The patient determines the contraceptive method of choice. Counseling should be tailored to them. Transmasculine patients on testosterone may have questions regarding how testosterone affects contraception, however, no research presently exists on how side effect profiles of contraceptive methods may be altered [47, 48]. Patients on testosterone should be informed of this when describing known effects and side effects of contraceptive methods (e.g., effects on uterine bleeding or cramps). Transmasculine patients may have additional concerns or goals regarding contraception beyond typical questions for cisgender females [47, 48]. There are a number of examples of these. However, every patient is unique and should be asked about their goals and concerns and should not be assumed based on gender.

First, some patients may experience distress related to gender dysphoria when discussing contraception or pregnancy [51]. Second, dysphoria associated with reproductive anatomy and physiology or a history of trauma or assault may impact their preference regarding methods for use [47]. Additionally, some patients may be

Table 8.2 Types of contraception and menstrual suppression

Hormonal contraception	Nonhormonal contraception	Noncontraceptive menstrual suppression
Estrogen and progestin	– Copper intrauterine device	– Progesterone pills
– Combined oral	– Fertility awareness methods	(Norethindrone, Provera)
contraceptive pills	– Condoms (internal and external)	– Danazol
– Transdermal patch	– Spermicide sponge	– Gonadotropin-releasing
– Vaginal ring	– Creams, foams, and	hormone agonists
Progestin	suppositories	– Selective estrogen receptor
– Progestin only pills	– Diaphragm	modulators
– Depot	– Sterilization (tubal ligation or	– Selective progestin receptor
Medroxyprogesterone	bilateral oophorectomy)	modulators
– Etonogestrel subdermal		– Aromatase inhibitors
implant		– Nonsteroidal anti-
– Levonorgestrel		inflammatory drugs[a]
intrauterine device		– Tranexamic acid[a]
	Hysterectomy	

[a]Menstrual reduction, not suppression

interested in or actively attempting to conceive, so pregnancy intention screening should be offered. Clinicians should be sensitive to this and support the patient's gender affirmation and utilize a trauma-informed approach throughout the decision-making process. Other examples of patient-centered considerations include concerns for needing an invasive pelvic exam, potential for chest tenderness, privacy or concealability of the method, frequent dosing, and the need for a clinician to discontinue the method [48]. A patient who has privacy concerns may prefer an etonogestrel implant or IUD, while a person who wants to self-discontinue if they dislike the method might not. A person who wants to avoid an invasive pelvic exam might prefer a pill, transdermal patch, or vaginal ring. At the same time, those may be preferable for someone worried about the potential for chest tenderness due to estrogen. Patients may also desire to avoid any estrogen-containing methods or any hormonal method altogether.

Any person utilizing an estrogen-containing method should be counseled on the increased risk of venous thromboembolism (VTE). Present data do not show an increased risk of VTE in transmasculine persons on testosterone [52]. Counseling should be as per cisgender female guidelines. Additionally, as there is no research on comorbidity risk stratification in transmasculine persons on testosterone using contraception, cisgender female guidelines regarding adverse outcomes should be employed [53].

Patients at risk for pregnancy should also be counseled on emergency contraception [54]. All methods should be offered, and guidelines do not presently have any contraindications for emergency contraception. There is no guidance on follow-up after emergency contraceptive use in transmasculine persons on testosterone. As patients may be amenorrheic, the typical guidance of monitoring for menstruation cannot be employed. Some recommend a follow-up pregnancy test 4 weeks after taking emergency contraception, particularly if there is any change in the patient's bleeding pattern or they experience new pelvic pain [48].

Genital Bleeding Workup and Management in Transmasculine Patients on Testosterone

Another referral to gynecologists is for genital bleeding on testosterone. Genital bleeding may occur from several sources [55]. Many of the causes of genital bleeding in persons not on testosterone can be seen in those on testosterone and should continue to be considered in the differential. In addition, there are testosterone-specific considerations that should also be included.

Testosterone-Specific Considerations in Genital Bleeding

First, vulvovaginal atrophy, which occurs in some patients on testosterone (see Sect. 8.2.3), can be a source of bleeding. Second, missed or low testosterone doses or withdrawal from a concomitant menstrual suppression therapy may cause uterine bleeding. Uterine bleeding due to missed doses is likely due to a drop in serum testosterone levels and the resulting endometrial and endogenous hormone effects. Some patients may be amenorrheic while on testosterone and concomitant hormone therapy (such as a contraceptive or puberty suppressing agent). Bleeding related to withdrawal of concomitant hormone therapy is likely due in part to the same reasons for bleeding following the withdrawal of similar medications in a person not on testosterone. For example, the loss of progestin action on the endometrial lining can induce endometrial shedding [56].

Unscheduled uterine bleeding may also occur on testosterone. While unscheduled bleeding is expected during low initial dosing, most patients achieve amenorrhea in the first year (85–100%) [57, 58]. Despite this, bleeding can occur even in persons achieving target range testosterone levels. In one study, 25% of transmasculine persons on testosterone who sought gender-affirming hysterectomies had bleeding at the time of presentation [8].

The reasons for unscheduled bleeding are unclear. In the multi-site hysterectomy pathology study, bleeding was not associated with thicker endometrial linings or a greater likelihood of proliferative activity (compared to inactive endometria) [8]. Endogenous hormone activity may affect bleeding risk but is difficult to assess clinically. While ovaries are suppressed in persons on testosterone they are not universally inactive [9, 14]. Estradiol is also in adipose tissue as a conversion from testosterone [59]. Past studies have not shown increased estradiol levels with increasing serum testosterone, suggesting no linear relationship between them [60]. Serum estradiol levels in most studies appear well suppressed [57, 58]. It is also unclear how testosterone directly influences the endometrium as most research has theorized that changes seen are indirectly due to endogenous sex steroid suppression [61]. A study that evaluated endometrial androgen receptor patterns on testosterone, found the lowest concentration in the endometrial epithelium; it is unclear how this might relate to, or explain, uterine bleeding in some patients [11].

Finally, endometrial malignancy which may present as genital bleeding, can still occur in transmasculine persons on testosterone, though the risk does not appear increased relative to the general population [8].

Evaluation and Management of Testosterone-Specific Considerations of Bleeding

There is no standard guidance from the American College of Obstetrics and Gynecology (ACOG) or other national bodies regarding evaluating genital bleeding on testosterone. All causes of genital bleeding should be considered on the differential.

In taking a history potential testosterone-related causes should be assessed through discussion of any vulvovaginal concerns, any missed or incorrect testosterone dosing, as well as recent changes in dosing or type of testosterone. Additional questions should be asked about any new hormonal method initiations, discontinuations, or dosing changes. Included in the gynecologic exam (Sect. 8.1) should be an assessment of estrogenization of the external genitalia (particularly if vulvovaginal atrophy is the suspected cause) [62]. Laboratory testing may include serum testosterone levels, particularly if concerns for missed or low doses or recent dosing changes. Serum estradiol and gonadotropins can be considered as well to evaluate for endogenous suppression or elevated estradiol levels.

If vulvovaginal atrophy is suspected, management is reviewed in Sect. 8.9. Patients with bleeding resulting from repeated missed doses may benefit from an alternate, longer-acting approach to testosterone, such as subcutaneous pellet therapy [63]. Those who are stopping concomitant hormonal medication should be counseled that this may induce a withdrawal bleed.

Once other sources are ruled out, unscheduled bleeding is the remaining uterine cause. Of note, transgender care guidelines recommend allowing up to 1 year after initiation of testosterone therapy to achieve amenorrhea due to variability in dosing protocols and baseline physiology (or 6–12 months of testosterone levels in the male range (320–1000 ng/dl)) [23]. Increasing testosterone when able and when desired by the patient is a first-line approach to the management of unscheduled bleeding. Despite this, some patients will continue to bleed (of note, menstrual suppression is a common goal for transmasculine patients seeking medical gender affirmation, either before, or as a part of initiating, testosterone. If patients desire more rapid menstrual suppression prior to the 1 year mark they should be offered it) [25, 64].

There are a number of regimens that can be offered for menstrual suppression (Table 8.2). There is presently no data on the superiority of any one method. Just as with contraception methods in Sect. 8.7, the method chosen should be tailored to the patient's goals. Nonhormonal medications (nonsteroidal anti-inflammatory drugs and tranexamic acid) may help reduce the amount of bleeding but are generally not successful at inducing amenorrhea [65, 66]. The most common methods of menstrual suppression are hormonal medications. Patients should be counseled that no data presently exists on the amenorrhea rate of any one method when taken with testosterone, and that amenorrhea cannot be guaranteed. Estrogen and progestin combined methods, progestin-only methods, and gonadotropin-releasing agonists are all available and not contraindicated in persons on testosterone. Danazol is an androgen-like medication previously used for endometriosis with resultant high amenorrhea rates [67]. It can be used alongside testosterone as a possible menstrual suppression method. Selective estrogen receptor modulators (SERM) have been discussed as a menstrual suppression agent [64]. However, present gynecologic guidelines recommend that any new uterine bleeding on a SERM be evaluated by endometrial sampling, which is invasive [68]. This should be included in the counseling of patients on their use and may not be a prioritized method. Some clinicians have used aromatase inhibitors for the management of unscheduled bleeding under the theory that bleeding is related to the peripheral conversion of androgens to estrogens via aromatase. However, no data has been published on the success of this method, and early studies do not support aromatase activity as a consistent etiology for elevated estrogen levels in persons on testosterone [69]. Selective progesterone receptor modulators have been shown in cisgender females to induce amenorrhea with use [70]. However, they are often only used for limited periods and are not universally available.

Surgical management of uterine bleeding includes ablation and hysterectomy [55]. Ablation is not reversible, will cause the uterus to be sterile, and is not a form of contraception. In cisgender females, it does not maintain prolonged amenorrhea with only 13–55% having amenorrhea 1 year following the procedure with decreasing efficacy at 5 years [71]. Hysterectomy may be desired by some patients experiencing unscheduled bleeding, though not all. The procedure should be offered to those who are interested. See Sect. 8.3 for more information regarding hysterectomy.

Vulvovaginal Atrophy

In patients where vulvovaginal atrophy is suspected as the source of bleeding, many of the same therapies and protocols used in postmenopausal cisgender women can be considered [72]. Vaginal moisturizers and lubricants (e.g., petroleum jelly) can be used. Local estrogen can also be considered, which includes pills, creams, and rings. Patients should be counseled that local estrogen use is not significantly absorbed in the uterus or systemically and will not impact testosterone's systemic virilization effects [73].

Pelvic Pain in Transmasculine Patients

Pelvic pain can occur in transmasculine patients. Masculinizing hormone therapy and gender-affirming surgeries can influence this. There may also be psychological and social factors that can influence their risk for, or management of, pain. Just as in cisgender persons, transmasculine persons can have multifaceted pelvic pain (e.g., influenced by gynecologic, urologic, gastroenterological, psychologic, dermatologic, musculoskeletal, or neurologic conditions). There is little evidence on how the pelvic pain evaluation differs in a transmasculine patient compared to a cisgender patient, but existing literature will be addressed here.

Psychological and Social Considerations in Pelvic Pain in Transmasculine Patients

Transmasculine patients may have certain experiences that influence their differential diagnosis of pelvic pain. For example, bathroom safety issues may influence bladder habits of transmasculine patients and may increase the frequency of voiding dysfunction or urinary tract infections [74]. Trauma is associated with chronic pain

8 Non-procreative Reproductive Issues and Sexual Function in Transmasculine...   121

in the larger population, and transgender patients experience many types of trauma (post-traumatic stress disorder (PTSD), intimate partner violence, abuse, and sexual assault) at high rates [2]. Transmasculine patients may also delay presentation for pain-related syndromes, due to a feeling of needing to suppress expressions of pain due to the social need to be perceived as masculine [75].

Testosterone-Related Considerations in Pelvic Pain in Transmasculine Patients

While no masculinizing therapy-related changes have been directly linked to pelvic pain, a pilot study identified a cohort of transmasculine persons who endorsed new-onset abdominopelvic pain after testosterone initiation [76]. There are a few potential etiologies for this related to physiologic changes from testosterone.

Uterine pain may be a possibility though it remains of unclear etiology. Some on testosterone complain of uterine cramping with or without bleeding, worsening when taking testosterone, or after orgasm [76]. Testosterone affects the uterus in certain ways, which may contribute to pelvic pain. For example, some persons still bleed while on testosterone and dysmenorrhea, or pain associated with menstruation may be a source [8]. Additionally, endometriosis has been found in patients on testosterone, further supporting that endometrial pain-related syndromes are possible, even in the setting of amenorrhea [13]. There are no studies that document an increase in the frequency of leiomyomata or adenomyosis when taking testosterone. Despite this, both have been found in persons taking testosterone and should continue to be considered in the differential [8]. Androgen receptors, as discussed earlier, have different patterns of expression in persons on testosterone compared to cisgender females, but how this might contribute to pain is unknown [11]. Known sources of ovarian pain do not appear increased in frequency on testosterone. Despite this, masses and cysts common to reproductive age cisgender women have been documented in transmasculine individuals on testosterone and should continue to be included in the differential [14]. Ovulation-related pain should decrease in frequency on testosterone, as data shows ovulation is mostly suppressed [9]. Vulvovaginal atrophy on testosterone as described in Sect. 8.2 can contribute to general pelvic pain and dyspareunia. Enlargement of the clitorophallus is a known effect of testosterone [25]. This can contribute to increased sensitivity, which can be pleasurable for some but may cause distress or pain due to a sustained erection.

There are few other causes presently known to arise from testosterone related to pelvic pain. Due to changes in muscle composition, testosterone may influence the abdominal wall and pelvic floor which can contribute to pelvic pain or dyspareunia [23]. While testosterone may be associated with increased bladder capacity and post-void residual volume, this may be more related to lifestyle changes (e.g., bladder habits due to bathroom safety concerns) than direct androgen-related changes [20]. Vulvovaginal atrophy is known to contribute to urinary tract infection frequency in cisgender women, however, this has not yet been documented in transmasculine persons on testosterone [21].

Masculinizing Genital Affirmation Surgery Considerations in Pelvic Pain in Transmasculine patients

Some transmasculine patients may undergo a hysterectomy, which carries the same risk for postoperative pain as hysterectomies done in cisgender women. Postoperative pain from changes in ligamentous support and pelvic floor is well documented in cisgender women. It is likely a risk in transmasculine individuals, particularly those who have not undergone vaginectomy [77].

Immediate postoperative pain sources following metoidioplasty and phalloplasty may include wound breakdown, flap loss, hematomas, and infection [28, 32]. Long-term causes of pain postoperatively can include granulation tissue, scarring, or strictures. Neo-urethral-related pain can include strictures, hair granulomas, or fistulas. Infections or lesions which may occur at the donor site can still occur in the donor tissue. For those who undergo testicular implants concomitant with these procedures, the implants can become infected, migrate or erode, and present with pain localized to the implants' area [33]. Erectile rods may be placed in the neophallus for erectile capacity, which can become infected or erode, and cause pain at the pubic bone due to pressure [34].

Evaluation and Management Considerations of Pelvic Pain in Transmasculine Patients

Pelvic pain in the transmasculine patient is approached similarly to that of a cisgender female patient. Unless native anatomy has been surgically removed or neo anatomy added, all causes of pain which would have been considered prior to gender-affirming therapies should be included in the differential. The history and physical should proceed as per Sect. 8.1 with a few additional considerations. First, external genitalia should be evaluated for signs of atrophy. Second, any neo-genitalia should include a thorough skin exam (with clarification of donor site) and voiding history and evaluation for postoperative complications. Third, the pelvic floor should be assessed, including assessing prolapse in those who have had a hysterectomy but retain vagina. Finally, a pelvic ultrasound (transabdominal for those who are not comfortable with a transvaginal) should be utilized to exclude masses or as an alternative to bimanual exam if declined by the patient.

Management will be targeting the suspected etiology of pain. Most pain sources can be treated as per cisgender guidelines [e.g., vulvovaginal atrophy, pelvic floor dysfunction, prolapse, urinary tract infections in a native urethra (for neo-urethral issues see below)] [78]. Suspected uterine-related pain with or without bleeding can be managed using medications commonly used for dysmenorrhea, including non-steroidal anti-inflammatory medications, estrogen and progestin combination contraceptives, and progesterone medications [79]. Gonadotropin Hormone Releasing analogs and danazol, and aromatase inhibitors can also be considered, particularly if there is concomitant bleeding or a concern for endometriosis [67, 79, 80]. Some may desire a hysterectomy; these patients should be counseled on the possibility that a hysterectomy is permanent yet may not resolve their pain [76].

If clitorophallus growth is the source of pain patients can try to change clothing and minimize contact with the sources that appear to induce arousal. If spontaneous, topical lidocaine may be tried or barrier methods (e.g., petroleum jelly). Centrally acting neuromodulating medications such as gabapentin or pregabalin can also be considered [81].

Regarding neogenitalia, most postoperative concerns (e.g., granulation tissue and scar formation) should be addressed by the original surgeon or one competent in masculinizing genital surgery. Any urinary concerns of a neo-urethra should be addressed by a urologist who performs these procedures. For STI-related pain, see Sect. 8.6. Management of any dermatologic concerns of the neophallus should be treated as they would for the donor site.

Conclusion

The transmasculine patient's gynecologic care encompasses a broad spectrum, including preventative health, sexual health, and surgical care, and pathologies such as pelvic pain or genital bleeding. While foundational approaches to evaluation and management are based on cisgender female guidelines for many of these areas, transmasculine gynecologic health nuances should be understood to ensure comprehensive and culturally competent care is provided. As the field continues to grow, a better understanding will follow of how to best tailor the approaches to gynecologic care for transmasculine patients, particularly for those on testosterone.

References

1. Raja S, Hasnain M, Hoersch M, Gove-Yin S, Rajagopalan C. Trauma informed care in medicine: current knowledge and future research directions. Fam Community Health. 2015;38(3):216–26.
2. James SE, Herman JL, Keisling M, Mottet L, Anafi M. The report of the 2015 US transgender survey. Washington, DC: National Center for Transgender Equality; 2016.
3. Defreyne J, Elaut E, Kreukels B, Fisher AD, Castellini G, Staphorsius A, et al. Sexual desire changes in transgender individuals upon initiation of hormone treatment: results from the longitudinal European network for the investigation of gender incongruence. J Sex Med. 2020;17(4):812–25.
4. Copen CE, Chandra A, Febo-Vazquez I. Sexual behavior, sexual attraction, and sexual orientation among adults aged 18-44 in the United States: data from the 2011-2013 National Survey of family growth. Natl Health Stat Rep. 2016;88:1–14.
5. Tree-McGrath CAF, Puckett JA, Reisner SL, Pantalone DW. Sexuality and gender affirmation in transgender men who have sex with cisgender men. Int J Transgender. 2018;19(4):389–400.
6. Fausto-Sterling A. Sexing the body: gender politics and the construction of sexuality. New York: Basic Books; 2000.

7. Bates CK, Carroll N, Potter J. The challenging pelvic examination. J Gen Intern Med. 2011;26(6):651–7.
8. Grimstad FW, Fowler KG, New EP, Ferrando CA, Pollard RR, Chapman G, et al. Uterine pathology in transmasculine persons on testosterone: a retrospective multicenter case series. Am J Obstet Gynecol. 2018.
9. Taub RL, Ellis SA, Neal-Perry G, Magaret AS, Prager SW, Micks EA. The effect of testosterone on ovulatory function in transmasculine individuals. Am J Obstet Gynecol. 2020.
10. Simitsidellis I, Saunders PTK, Gibson DA. Androgens and endometrium: new insights and new targets. Mol Cell Endocrinol. 2018;15(465):48–60.
11. Loverro G, Resta L, Dellino M, Edoardo DN, Cascarano MA, Loverro M, et al. Uterine and ovarian changes during testosterone administration in young female-to-male transsexuals. Taiwan J Obstet Gynecol. 2016;55(5):686–91.
12. Khalifa MA, Toyama A, Klein ME, Santiago V. Histologic features of hysterectomy specimens from female-male transgender individuals. Int J Gynecol Pathol. 2018;
13. Shim JY, Laufer MR, Grimstad FW. Dysmenorrhea and endometriosis in transgender adolescents. J Pediatr Adolesc Gynecol. 2020 Oct;33(5):524–8.
14. Grimstad FW, Fowler KG, New EP, Ferrando CA, Pollard RR, Chapman G, et al. Ovarian histopathology in transmasculine persons on testosterone: a multicenter case series. J Sex Med. 2020;17(9):1807–18.
15. Ikeda K, Baba T, Noguchi H, Nagasawa K, Endo T, Kiya T, et al. Excessive androgen exposure in female-to-male transsexual persons of reproductive age induces hyperplasia of the ovarian cortex and stroma but not polycystic ovary morphology. Hum Reprod. 2013;28(2):453–61.
16. Lierman S, Tilleman K, Braeckmans K, Peynshaert K, Weyers S, T'Sjoen G, et al. Fertility preservation for trans men: frozen-thawed in vitro matured oocytes collected at the time of ovarian tissue processing exhibit normal meiotic spindles. J Assist Reprod Genet. 2017;34(11):1449–56.
17. Light AD, Obedin-Maliver J, Sevelius JM, Kerns JL. Transgender men who experienced pregnancy after female-to-male gender transitioning. Obstet Gynecol. 2014;124(6):1120–7.
18. Winston McPherson G, Long T, Salipante SJ, Rongitsch JA, Hoffman NG, Stephens K, et al. The vaginal microbiome of transgender men. Clin Chem. 2019;65(1):199–207.
19. Fisher AD, Castellini G, Ristori J, Casale H, Cassioli E, Sensi C, et al. Cross-sex hormone treatment and psychobiological changes in transsexual persons: two-year follow-up data. J Clin Endocrinol Metab. 2016;101(11):4260–9.
20. Matsuo K, Ichihara K, Gotoh M, Masumori N. Comparison of the uroflowmetry parameter results between transgender males undergoing gender-affirming hormone therapy and age-matched cisgender females: preliminary data. Transgend Health. 2019;4(1):152–6.
21. Raz R. Urinary tract infection in postmenopausal women. Korean J Urol. 2011;52(12):801–8.
22. Grimstad F, Boskey E. Empowering transmasculine youth by enhancing reproductive health counseling in the primary care setting. J Adolesc Health. 2020;66(6):653–5.
23. UCSF Transgender Care, Department of Family and Community Medicine, University of California San Francisco. Guidelines for the Primary and Gender-Affirming Care of Transgender and Gender Nonbinary People [Internet]. 2nd ed. Deutsch MB, ed; 2016. Available from: transcare.ucsf.edu/guidelines.
24. Reilly ZP, Fruhauf TF, Martin SJ. Barriers to evidence-based transgender care: knowledge gaps in gender-affirming hysterectomy and oophorectomy. Obstet Gynecol. 2019;134(4):714–7.
25. Hembree WC, Cohen-Kettenis PT, Gooren L, Hannema SE, Meyer WJ, Murad MH, et al. Endocrine treatment of gender-dysphoric/gender-incongruent persons: an endocrine society clinical practice guideline. J Clin Endocrinol Metab. 2017;102(11):3869–903.
26. Nahata L, Chen D, Moravek MB, Quinn GP, Sutter ME, Taylor J, et al. Understudied and underreported: fertility issues in transgender youth—a narrative review. J Pediatr. 2019;205:265–71.
27. Evans EC, Matteson KA, Orejuela FJ, Alperin M, Balk EM, El-Nashar S, et al. Salpingo-oophorectomy at the time of benign hysterectomy: a systematic review. Obstet Gynecol. 2016;128(3):476–85.

8 Non-procreative Reproductive Issues and Sexual Function in Transmasculine...

28. Frey JD, Poudrier G, Chiodo MV, Hazen A. A systematic review of metoidioplasty and radial forearm flap phalloplasty in female-to-male transgender genital reconstruction: is the "ideal" neophallus an achievable goal? Plast Reconstr Surg Glob Open. 2016;4(12):e1131.
29. Djordjevic ML, Stojanovic B, Bizic M. Metoidioplasty: techniques and outcomes. Transl Androl Urol. 2019;8(3):248–53.
30. Morrison SD, Shakir A, Vyas KS, Kirby J, Crane CN, Lee GK. Phalloplasty: a review of techniques and outcomes. Plast Reconstr Surg. 2016;138(3):594–615.
31. Heston AL, Esmonde NO, Dugi DD, Berli JU. Phalloplasty: techniques and outcomes. Transl Androl Urol. 2019;8(3):254–65.
32. Remington AC, Morrison SD, Massie JP, Crowe CS, Shakir A, Wilson SC, et al. Outcomes after phalloplasty: do transgender patients and multiple urethral procedures carry a higher rate of complication? Plast Reconstr Surg. 2018;141(2):220e–9e.
33. Pigot GLS, Al-Tamimi M, Ronkes B, van der Sluis TM, Özer M, Smit JM, et al. Surgical outcomes of neoscrotal augmentation with testicular prostheses in transgender men. J Sex Med. 2019;16(10):1664–71.
34. van der Sluis WB, Pigot GLS, Al-Tamimi M, Ronkes BL, de Haseth KB, Özer M, et al. A retrospective cohort study on surgical outcomes of penile prosthesis implantation surgery in transgender men after phalloplasty. Urology. 2019;132:195–201.
35. James SE, Herman JL, Rankin S, Keisling M, Mottet M, Anafi M. The report of the 2015 U.S. transgender survey [internet]. Washington, DC: National Center for Transgender Equality; 2016. Available from: http://www.transequality.org/sites/default/files/docs/usts/USTS%20 Full%20Report%20-%20FINAL%201.6.17.pdf
36. Bluebond-Langner R, Berli JU, Sabino J, Chopra K, Singh D, Fischer B. Top surgery in transgender men: how far can you push the envelope? Plast Reconstr Surg. 2017;139(4):873e–82e.
37. Olson-Kennedy J, Warus J, Okonta V, Belzer M, Clark LF. Chest reconstruction and chest Dysphoria in transmasculine minors and young adults: comparisons of nonsurgical and post-surgical cohorts. JAMA Pediatr. 2018;172(5):431–6.
38. MacDonald T, Noel-Weiss J, West D, Walks M, Biener M, Kibbe A, et al. Transmasculine individuals' experiences with lactation, chestfeeding, and gender identity: a qualitative study. BMC Pregnancy Childbirth [Internet]. 2016 [cited 2020 Nov 4];16. Available from: https:// www.ncbi.nlm.nih.gov/pmc/articles/PMC4867534/
39. de Blok CJM, Wiepjes CM, Nota NM, van Engelen K, Adank MA, Dreijerink KMA, et al. Breast cancer risk in transgender people receiving hormone treatment: nationwide cohort study in the Netherlands. BMJ [Internet]. 2019; May 14 [cited 2019 Dec 1];365. Available from: https://www.bmj.com/content/365/bmj.l1652
40. Stowell JT, Grimstad FW, Kirkpatrick DL, Brown ER, Santucci RA, Crane C, et al. Imaging findings in transgender patients after gender-affirming surgery. Radiographics. 2019;39(5):1368–92.
41. Meites E, Szilagyi PG, Chesson HW, Unger ER, Romero JR, Markowitz LE. Human papillomavirus vaccination for adults: updated recommendations of the advisory committee on immunization practices. MMWR Morb Mortal Wkly Rep. 2019;68(32):698–702.
42. Adkins BD, Barlow AB, Jack A, Schultenover SJ, Desouki MM, Coogan AC, et al. Characteristic findings of cervical Papanicolaou tests from transgender patients on androgen therapy: challenges in detecting dysplasia. Cytopathology. 2018;29(3):281–7.
43. Bateson DJ, Weisberg E. An open-label randomized trial to determine the most effective regimen of vaginal estrogen to reduce the prevalence of atrophic changes reported in postmenopausal cervical smears. Menopause. 2009 Aug;16(4):765–9.
44. Huh WK, Ault KA, Chelmow D, Davey DD, Goulart RA, Garcia FAR, et al. Use of primary high-risk human papillomavirus testing for cervical cancer screening: interim clinical guidance. Obstet Gynecol. 2015 Feb;125(2):330–7.
45. Reisner SL, Deutsch MB, Peitzmeier SM, White Hughto JM, Cavanaugh TP, Pardee DJ, et al. Test performance and acceptability of self- versus provider-collected swabs for high-risk HPV DNA testing in female-to-male trans masculine patients. PLoS One. 2018;13(3):e0190172.

46. Workowski K, Bolan G. Centers for Disease Control and Prevention. Sexually Transmitted Diseases Treatment Guidelines [Internet]. 2015 p. 64(No. RR-3): 1–137. Available from: https://www.cdc.gov/std/tg2015/default.htm
47. Bonnington A, Dianat S, Kerns J, Hastings J, Hawkins M, De Haan G, et al. Society of Family Planning clinical recommendations: contraceptive counseling for transgender and gender diverse people who were female sex assigned at birth. Contraception. 2020;102(2):70–82.
48. Krempasky C, Harris M, Abern L, Grimstad F. Contraception across the transmasculine spectrum. Am J Obstet Gynecol. 2019.
49. Light A, Wang L-F, Zeymo A, Gomez-Lobo V. Family planning and contraception use in transgender men. Contraception. 2018;98(4):266–9.
50. Toxnet. Testosterone [Internet]. [cited 2019 Mar 2]. Available from: https://toxnet.nlm.nih.gov/cgi-bin/sis/search2/r?dbs+hsdb:@term+@DOCNO+3398
51. Hoffkling A, Obedin-Maliver J, Sevelius J. From erasure to opportunity: a qualitative study of the experiences of transgender men around pregnancy and recommendations for providers. BMC Pregnancy Childbirth. 2017;17(2):332.
52. Shatzel JJ, Connelly KJ, DeLoughery TG. Thrombotic issues in transgender medicine: a review. Am J Hematol. 2017;92(2):204–8.
53. Curtis KM. U.S. Medical eligibility criteria for contraceptive use, 2016. MMWR Recomm Rep. 2016, 65
54. Practice Bulletin Summary No. 152: emergency contraception. Obstet Gynecol. 2015 Sep;126(3):685–6.
55. American College of Obstetricians and Gynecologists. ACOG committee opinion no. 557: Management of acute abnormal uterine bleeding in nonpregnant reproductive-aged women. Obstet Gynecol. 2013;121(4):891–6.
56. Melmed S, Williams RH. Williams textbook of endocrinology. 12th ed. Shlomo Melmed, et al. Philadelphia: Elsevier/Saunders; 2011. xiv+1897.
57. Deutsch MB, Bhakri V, Kubicek K. Effects of cross-sex hormone treatment on transgender women and men. Obstet Gynecol. 2015;125(3):605–10.
58. Pelusi C, Costantino A, Martelli V, Lambertini M, Bazzocchi A, Ponti F, et al. Effects of three different testosterone formulations in female-to-male transsexual persons. J Sex Med. 2014;11(12):3002–11.
59. Siiteri PK. Adipose tissue as a source of hormones. Am J Clin Nutr. 1987;45(1 Suppl):277–82.
60. Morishima A, Grumbach MM, Simpson ER, Fisher C, Qin K. Aromatase deficiency in male and female siblings caused by a novel mutation and the physiological role of estrogens. J Clin Endocrinol Metab. 1995;80(12):3689–98.
61. American College of Obstetricians and Gynecologists' Committee on Practice Bulletins—Gynecology. ACOG Practice Bulletin No. 194: polycystic ovary syndrome. Obstet Gynecol. 2018;131(6):e157–71.
62. Unger CA. Care of the transgender patient: the role of the gynecologist. Am J Obstet Gynecol. 2014;210(1):16–26.
63. McCullough A. A review of testosterone pellets in the treatment of hypogonadism. Curr Sex Health Rep. 2014;6(4):265–9.
64. Carswell JM, Roberts SA. Induction and maintenance of amenorrhea in transmasculine and nonbinary adolescents. Transgend Health. 2017;2(1):195–201.
65. Matteson KA, Rahn DD, Wheeler TL, Casiano E, Siddiqui NY, Harvie HS, et al. Nonsurgical management of heavy menstrual bleeding: a systematic review. Obstet Gynecol. 2013;121(3):632–43.
66. Bryant-Smith AC, Lethaby A, Farquhar C, Hickey M. Antifibrinolytics for heavy menstrual bleeding. Cochrane Database Syst Rev [Internet] 2018 [cited 2020 Dec 5];(4). https://doi.org/10.1002/14651858.CD000249.pub2/full
67. Rose GL, Dowsett M, Mudge JE, White JO, Jeffcoate SL. The inhibitory effects of danazol, danazol metabolites, gestrinone, and testosterone on the growth of human endometrial cells in vitro. Fertil Steril. 1988;49(2):224–8.

68. Committee Opinion No. 601: Tamoxifen and uterine cancer. Obstet Gynecol. 2014;123(6):1394–7.
69. Chan KJ, Jolly D, Liang JJ, Weinand JD, Safer JD. Estrogen levels do not rise with testosteroen treatment for transgender men. Endocr Pract. 2018;24(4):329–33.
70. Donnez J, Tatarchuk TF, Bouchard P, Puscasiu L, Zakharenko NF, Ivanova T, et al. Ulipristal acetate versus placebo for fibroid treatment before surgery. N Engl J Med. 2012;366(5):409–20.
71. ACOG Committee on Practice Bulletins. ACOG practice bulletin. Clinical management guidelines for obstetrician-gynecologists. Number 81, May 2007. Obstet Gynecol. 2007 May;109(5):1233–48.
72. Moulder J, Carrillo J, Carey E. Pelvic pain in the transgender man. Curr Obstet Gynecol Rep. 2020.
73. Bachmann G, Bouchard C, Hoppe D, Ranganath R, Altomare C, Vieweg A, et al. Efficacy and safety of low-dose regimens of conjugated estrogens cream administered vaginally. Menopause. 2009;16(4):719–27.
74. Hardacker CT, Baccellieri A, Mueller ER, Brubaker L, Hutchins G, Zhang JLY, et al. Bladder health experiences, perceptions and knowledge of sexual and gender minorities. Int J Environ Res Public Health [Internet]. 2019 [cited 2020 Dec 6];16(17). Available from: https://www.ncbi.nlm.nih.gov/pmc/articles/PMC6747507/
75. Detloff M. Gender please, without the gender police: rethinking pain in archetypal narratives of butch, transgender, and FTM masculinity. J Lesbian Stud. 2006;10(1–2):87–105.
76. Grimstad FW, Boskey E, Grey M. New-onset abdominopelvic pain after initiation of testosterone therapy among trans-masculine persons: a community-based exploratory survey. LGBT Health. 2020;7(5):248–53.
77. Brandsborg B, Nikolajsen L, Hansen CT, Kehlet H, Jensen TS. Risk factors for chronic pain after hysterectomy: a nationwide questionnaire and database study. Anesthesiology. 2007;106(5):1003–12.
78. Yang CC, Miller JL, Omidpanah A, Krieger JN. Physical examination for men and women with urological chronic pelvic pain syndromes: a MAPP network study. Urology. 2018;116:23–9.
79. ACOG Committee Opinion No. 760: Dysmenorrhea and endometriosis in the adolescent. Obstet Gynecol. 2018 Dec;132(6):e249–58.
80. Ferrero S, Gillott DJ, Venturini PL, Remorgida V. Use of aromatase inhibitors to treat endometriosis-related pain symptoms: a systematic review. Reprod Biol Endocrinol. 2011 Jun;21(9):89.
81. American College of Obstetricians and Gynecologists' Committee on Gynecologic Practice, American Society for Colposcopy and Cervical Pathology (ASCCP). Committee opinion No 673: persistent vulvar pain. Obstet Gynecol. 2016;128(3):e78–84.

Chapter 9
Non-procreative Reproductive Issues and Sexual Function in Transfeminine Individuals

Kyle R. Latack, Shane D. Morrison, and Miriam Hadj-Moussa

The number of individuals seeking gender-affirming medical and surgical services is increasing. These modalities aim to reduce gender dysphoria caused by gender incongruence in transgender and non-binary (TGNB) individuals. While this distress alone can impact sexual health, so can medical and surgical interventions. This chapter aims to provide a discussion of the non-procreative reproductive issues and sexual function in transfeminine individuals before, during, and after gender-affirming treatments. An understanding of sexual health in this population is crucial to improving quality of life and adequately counseling individuals on the impact of the available gender-affirming treatments.

Overview of Sexual Function

In order to discuss non-procreative reproductive issues in transfeminine individuals, it is necessary to establish a framework for sexual health and sexual dysfunction. The World Health Organization defines sexual health as a "state of physical, emotional, mental, and social well-being in relation to sexuality; it is not merely the

---

K. R. Latack
Keck School of Medicine of the University of Southern California, Los Angeles, CA, USA

Department of Obstetrics and Gynecology, University of Michigan, Ann Arbor, USA

S. D. Morrison
Section of Plastic Surgery, University of Michigan, Ann Arbor, MI, USA

Department of Plastic Surgery, Seattle Children's Hospital, Seattle, USA
e-mail: shanedm@med.umich.edu

M. Hadj-Moussa (✉)
Department of Urology, University of Michigan, Ann Arbor, MI, USA
e-mail: mhadjmou@med.umich.edu

© The Author(s), under exclusive license to Springer Nature
Switzerland AG 2023
M. B. Moravek, G. de Haan (eds.), *Reproduction in Transgender and Nonbinary Individuals*, https://doi.org/10.1007/978-3-031-14933-7_9

absence of disease, dysfunction, or infirmity" [1]. Sexuality and sexual well-being are multimodal being impacted by biological, psychological, and sociological factors. Understanding each of these components, as well as how they intersect, is important for improving sexual health.

Sexual Activity and Orientation in Transfeminine Individuals

Transfeminine individuals express the whole spectrum of sexual orientations, including those that are fluid and those that change during gender-related treatments. A recent study reports that 91% of transfeminine individuals not seeking gender affirmation and 88% after gender affirmation have been sexually active [2]. Within the same study, 58% of those not seeking gender affirmation reported sexual activity within the last 6 months. An identified area of distress for transfeminine individuals is finding partners, and being in a relationship was correlated with increased sexual satisfaction.

When it comes to sexual practices, transfeminine individuals prior to surgery may desire to avoid using their natal genitals. One study found that only half of untreated transfeminine individuals engage their genitals in sexual activity and 15% derive pleasure from involving genitals [3]. Sexual function does not solely rely on a partner though as transfeminine individuals report masturbating with a reported rate of 72–78% [4]. The frequency of masturbation can be utilized as a measurement of sexual desire and a way to track changes during treatment course.

Important Considerations

Assessing Sexual Desire and Function

Given the complex nature of sexual desire and function, there are many considerations when approaching non-procreative reproductive issues in transfeminine individuals and evaluating research on the topic. To start, at this time there are no validated questionnaires to evaluate treatment outcomes in the TGNB population [5]. Tools such as the Female Sexual Function Index (FSFI) are common in the literature though they were developed in cisgender populations and particularly those in heterosexual relationships. At best, they may serve as a proxy or an approximant. Additionally, research participants are typically heterogenous often mixing individuals who either desire and/or have received different treatments for their gender affirmation. With such heterogenicity in the study populations, it may be difficult to draw conclusions from the data. Studies also often focus on individuals prior to planned surgery or following surgery, which is not representative of the entire transfeminine population.

Psychological Health

TGNB individuals, and particularly those who identify as transfeminine, are at a high risk of psychological, physical, and sexual abuse [6]. This increased risk can dramatically impact sexual desire and function. A history of abuse, as well as stigma and discrimination, can also contribute to the increased prevalence of depression in the transgender community. While depression alone can impact sexual health, the pharmacologic treatments also notably have undesired sexual side effects. All of these factors are important considerations when optimizing sexual health. A thorough sexual history is warranted with a focus not only on psychosocial aspects, but also the patient's sexual goals and desires.

Sexually Transmitted Infections

An additional concern when discussing non-procreative reproductive issues is sexually transmitted infection (STI) prevalence. HIV and other STIs more commonly affect transfeminine individuals than cisgender women. Proposed reasons have included higher rates of unprotected anal intercourse, multiple sexual partners, or being involved in sex work. Other contextual factors may be involved, such as mental health issues, physical abuse, and inequalities in healthcare, among others [7]. Healthcare providers should ensure adequate discussion about STI prevention while also being mindful of social contexts that may increase risk. Notably, research on STIs in the TGNB population makes up a large portion of the literature on sexual health in the TGNB population with less data on noninfectious sexual health concerns [6]. The remainder of this chapter will focus on non-procreative reproductive issues outside of STIs with specific attention to the current stage an individual is at in treatment.

Pre-treatment

In this section, the focus will be on individuals who identify as transfeminine but have not undergone any medical or surgical treatments. While this subgroup represents a sizeable proportion of those who identify as transfeminine, there is a paucity of evidence-based research focused on individuals prior to treatment. Instead, research has typically focused on sexual function in individuals undergoing (or who have completed) treatment.

When assessing an individual pre-treatment, it is important to distinguish between those who do not desire treatments versus individuals who desire and are currently waiting to undergo treatment (i.e., unfulfilled treatment desire); though studies may not always make this distinction. Within the treatment timeline, both non-treated and undertreated individuals represent an important group of individuals as there is a limited number of providers adequately trained to provide gender-focused care. Oftentimes individuals face barriers including insurance and geography as they may need to travel to find a qualified physician. Additionally, there may be long wait times to establish an initial appointment once a physician is identified. Understanding the sexual health desires and needs of this group is important as 28% of transfeminine individuals with unmet health needs report sexual dissatisfaction though 47% report sex as important or very important [2].

Sexual Desire

An initial aspect of sexual health is sexual desire. Desire refers to the urge, drive, or lust that motivates sexual activity. For individuals in the pre-treatment stage, sexual desire is impacted by psychological and sociological factors within sexuality. Transfeminine individuals report a high prevalence of depression and anxiety which can negatively impact sexual desire and arousal. Additionally, this population reports dissatisfaction with body image and their sexual experiences in general.

A recent study of 307 transfeminine individuals through the European Network for the Investigation of Gender Incongruence (ENGI) sought to identify the prevalence of sexual dysfunction in this population. Within the no-treatment group, 40% of participants reported difficulties in initiating and seeking sexual contacts [8]. This is in contrast to only 14.3% of participants reporting low sexual desire and 18.8% reporting too strong of sexual desire. For some transfeminine individuals, low sexual desire may be present but not viewed as stressful given the presence of other factors such as fear of sexual contacts and aversion to sexual activity [4]. This may be particularly true in those with unfulfilled treatment.

One possible method for examining sexual behavior quantitively is through masturbation frequency. In one analysis, a significantly higher percentage of transfeminine individuals who did not desire treatment reported masturbating than those with unfulfilled and fulfilled treatment. Additionally, this group also reported a higher frequency of masturbation [2]. When the authors examined factors associated with frequency of sex, they found that having unfulfilled treatment desires was associated with a lower frequency of sex compared to fulfilled treatment desires. Regardless of the group, body satisfaction was found to be a predictor of the frequency of sex.

Sexual Function

When examining sexual function, a distinction can be made between sexual arousal and reaching orgasm. Additional issues related to sexual function are satisfaction and dyspareunia. Transfeminine persons may experience distress arising from these aspects of their sexual health.

Arousal Sexual arousal includes the subjective feeling of being aroused as well as the physiological response. For transfeminine individuals who have not undergone treatment, a desired physiologic response may be the ability to achieve and maintain an erection. It is important to note, however, that not all individuals desire to involve their phallus during sexual encounters.

For transfeminine individuals who have not undergone treatment, 33% reported difficulties getting sexually aroused which was significantly higher than those who underwent vaginoplasty [8]. Multiple factors may play a role in this including the reported difficulties initiating and seeking sexual contacts, aversion against sexual activity, and fear of sexual contacts.

Prior to medical treatment (surgical and non-surgical), transfeminine individuals display similar brain activation patterns during sexual arousal as cisgender women [9]. However, the sexual orientation of subjects in this study was mixed and there was no study of physiologic sexual arousal.

Orgasm Orgasm represents the highest point of sexual arousal, however, transfeminine individuals report difficulties achieving an orgasm. In Kerckhof et al. [8], almost 47% of individuals who have not received treatment report difficulties in achieving an orgasm. This may be due to difficulties in achieving/maintaining an erection as well as other psychosocial factors as described above.

Pain Even prior to surgery or other treatments, transfeminine individuals report dyspareunia. In one study, transfeminine individuals who were pre-treatment reported pain during intercourse at levels similar to after surgery; 29% versus 27%, respectively [8]. In the same group, 31% of participants who had not undergone treatment reported pain after intercourse. The source of pain in this population is unclear and could be the result of either the nature of sexual activities (such as anal penetrative sex) or due to increased pelvic floor dysfunction. Even prior to surgery, transfeminine individuals are reported to have high rates of pelvic floor dysfunction (42%) and those with a history of abuse had an even higher rate [10]. The exact cause of pelvic floor dysfunction is unclear, but psychological factors, including history of abuse, can exacerbate such dysfunction. Some transfeminine individuals may utilize genital "tucking" practices which may damage skin integrity but likely do not contribute to the pelvic floor dysfunction seen in this population.

Hormone Therapy

For transfeminine individuals, the goal of hormone therapy is to suppress androgens and increase estrogen levels to those found in premenopausal, mid-cycle, and cisgender females. Current treatments include exogenous estrogen and anti-androgen therapy. A suppression in androgens can impact sexual desire as well as function through a decrease in spontaneous and nocturnal erections, cessation of semen production, and decreased ejaculate volumes. As noted in the previous section, not all transfeminine individuals on hormone therapy will wish to involve their genitals in sexual activity. Therefore, the unique desires and needs of each patient must be elucidated through a thoughtful sexual history.

Sexual Desire

It is generally described that a decrease in androgens leads to a decrease in sexual desire, though the relationship between sex hormones and desire is complex. In fact, testosterone therapy is a treatment for hypoactive sexual desire dysfunction in perimenopausal and postmenopausal cisgender women. For transfeminine individuals undergoing hormonal therapy, sexual desire may fluctuate throughout the course of hormone therapy.

To better elucidate the changes during hormone therapy, Defreyne et al. [11] conducted a prospective study through the ENGI protocol with cross-sectional assessments at baseline, month three, 1 year, and 3 years comparing changes in desire between transfeminine and transmasculine individuals. This study found that at 3 months, transfeminine individuals had a significantly lower desire score than both their baseline and transmasculine individuals at the same time point. Notably, however, at 3 years of treatment, transfeminine individuals actually had a significantly higher score than their baseline whereas such change was not seen in transmasculine individuals. This study also noted that undergoing gonadectomy was associated with increased sexual desire in both transmasculine and transfeminine individuals; though the opposite effect is seen in the cisgender population. The authors discuss how the differences in motivation for undergoing gonadectomy may contribute to this difference. Such results are not surprising as individuals who progress through treatments report higher body satisfaction.

As noted above, a lack of sexual desire may not cause distress. The transient decrease in sexual desire when starting hormone therapy may be welcomed in women awaiting affirming surgery especially if they have aversion to sexual activity. The idea of progressing through treatment may also be assuring and limiting distress. One study reports that starting hormone therapy decreased distress even if desire is impacted [12] thus highlighting the role of psychosocial well-being in overall sexual health.

Given the relationship between testosterone and sexual desire, testosterone replacement has been proposed for individuals with low desire. Data supporting this hypothesis are present in one retrospective study, though the authors studied transfeminine individuals who underwent surgery as well [13]. The impact of such replacement prior to surgery, either in individuals waiting or those who do not desire surgery, is unclear. Perhaps the best way to improve sexual desire is by ensuring timely access to surgical care for individuals who desire it.

Sexual Function

Given that not all transfeminine individuals desire or can access genital surgery, the sexual function of an individual will vary based on their personal desires to utilize natal organs (e.g., penetration with their phallus).

Arousal For transfeminine individuals with a phallus and who desire the ability to penetrate, the arousal phase is marked by the ability to achieve and maintain an erection. The ability to achieve an erection is partially based on increased penile blood flow in a testosterone-dependent process. When examining erections in transfeminine individuals on anti-androgens, there was no difference in outcomes before and after hormonal treatment [14]. However, the authors noted a decrease in nocturnal erections. When examining prevalence of dysfunction regarding difficulties to get sexually aroused, 33% report difficulties getting sexually aroused [8]. Therefore, for transfeminine individuals who seek to maintain the ability to achieve an erection, low-dose testosterone or phosphodiesterase type 5 inhibitors may represent a viable treatment option.

Orgasm For transfeminine individuals who maintain their phallus, an orgasm leading to ejaculation can either be the goal or a source of distress. Low testosterone may cause ejaculatory difficulties while on hormone therapy. In fact, Kerckhof et al. [8] find that 29% of transfeminine individuals receiving hormone therapy report dysfunction in ability to achieve an orgasm. Another 15% report distress from the absence of an ejaculation. Conversely, 9% report distress from an unwanted ejaculation. This marked difference in the desired outcome highlights the importance of understanding an individual's sexual function goals as it cannot be assumed an orgasm with ejaculation is always desired.

Pain Transfeminine individuals receiving hormone therapy may experience pain during intercourse similarly to those individuals who have not received any treatment. In Kerckhof et al. [8], 11% of transfeminine individuals receiving hormone therapy report dysfunction from pain during intercourse, and another 9% report distress from pain after. Once again, the source of pain is unclear in this group. The authors hypothesize it is possibly due to more frequent anal penetration. Similar to transfeminine individuals who have not received any treatment, the pain could be related to pelvic floor dysfunction. When Jiang et al. [10] evaluated pelvic floor function in transfeminine individuals, all participants had received hormone therapy so an additional proposed mechanism may change due to hormone therapy. However, the relationship between hormone therapy and pelvic dysfunction is unclear. Estrogen plays a role in collagen metabolism in the pelvic floor and data shows that systemic estrogen therapy can actually worsen urinary incontinence [15].

Surgery

Though not all transfeminine individuals desire surgical treatment, for those who do, the results can greatly impact sexual health. This section will specifically examine the impact of genital surgery (as opposed to breast augmentation), though the increased body satisfaction following a breast augmentation may support an improvement in sexual health. For transfeminine individuals the key surgeries are:

orchiectomy, penectomy, clitoroplasty, labiaplasty, and the creation of a neovagina (vaginoplasty). An important surgical consideration that requires discussion with the patient is their desire for vaginal depth sufficient for vaginal intercourse. Not all individuals will desire such depth, however, for those who do, the goal of the vaginoplasty is to create a neovagina that allows for penetration with a neoclitoris that is sexually responsive. However, such procedures can require daily vaginal dilation which can serve as a source of stress for patients.

There are multiple options for the surgical approach to creating the neovagina and a more detailed explanation is beyond the scope of this chapter. Generally speaking, the most common is the penile skin inversion technique. Here, the skin of the penis and scrotum is inverted to form the vaginal wall and the neovagina is formed in the space in front of the rectum and behind the bladder/prostate. The glans penis is used for neoclitoris formation to preserve sensitivity and allow for orgasm. Within one study, the mean depth from this approach was 10–13.5 cm and a width of 3–4 cm. In this cohort, 75% of patients reported having vaginal intercourse and satisfaction was high [16].

Another approach is through a bowel vaginoplasty or peritoneal augmentation of the vaginal apex. Similar dimensions to the penile skin inversion technique are achieved as well as vaginal intercourse and satisfaction.

Desire Transfeminine individuals who have undergone surgical treatment may have enhanced sexual desire which may be due to increased body satisfaction. Compared to transfeminine individuals awaiting surgery, those who had undergone surgery reported higher sexual desire [4]. Following surgery, transfeminine individuals have a significantly lower prevalence of low sexual desire than those receiving hormonal therapy [8]. Additionally, the post-surgery group has a significantly lower prevalence of aversion against sexual activity compared to those receiving hormone therapy with a drop from 20% to 9%.

Following gender-affirming surgery, transfeminine people typically continue their hormone treatment. Given the prevalence of hypoactive sexual desire in this population, even following surgery, one proposed treatment may be testosterone replacement. One pilot study examined testosterone replacement in a group of transfeminine individuals after gender-affirming surgery and found a significant improvement in sexual desire [13] without noticeable side effects.

Arousal Transfeminine individuals after surgery report less difficulty with sexual arousal which may be related to increased body satisfaction. One study found the average time to first sexual arousal after surgery was 7.5 months [17]. This may be due to the physical process of recovery including general surgical pain as well as pain from dilation. Adapting to body changes and fear of injury may delay return of arousal. Additionally, surgeons may potentially impose restrictions on sexual activity during the recovery process which could also delay return of sexual arousal.

For transfeminine individuals who have undergone vaginoplasty, physiologic arousal can be represented through vaginal lubrication which has been shown to be possible [4]. However, this physiologic lubrication may not be sufficient for vaginal

9 Non-procreative Reproductive Issues and Sexual Function in Transfeminine... 137

penetrative intercourse. For individuals with a vagina, lack of lubrication can cause discomfort or pain during vaginal intercourse. Even within the cisgender population, 62% of women report ever using lubrication for vaginal intercourse and 25% report using it within the past month [18]. Kerckhof et al. [8] report a significantly higher prevalence of pain during sexual intercourse in transfeminine individuals after surgery compared to when only on hormone therapy. That level is similar to transfeminine individuals without treatment.

Arousal can also be measured objectively through either vaginal blood flow or functional MRI (fMRI) for brain activity patterns. Studies have found that transfeminine and cisgender individuals have similarities in objective arousal patterns, though transfeminine individuals may actually demonstrate higher concordance with subjective and objective arousal [4].

Additional measures of arousal using the FSFI have also been reported. Studies find that the majority of transfeminine experience sexual arousal with FSFI scores for arousal similar to cisgender women with sexual problems like low desire and pain [4].

Orgasm The question of whether transfeminine individuals are able to orgasm after vaginoplasty, and if so the quality of such orgasms, has been examined in multiple studies. It is reported that 62–100% of transfeminine individuals are able to reach orgasm after surgery [4]. However, difficulties achieving orgasm are still present and can cause distress. Following surgery, 29% of women still report difficulties achieving an orgasm [8].

There are also qualitative changes reported in the nature of orgasms in transfeminine individuals following surgery including more intense, smoother, longer, and more pleasurable [4]. It is important to note though that there may be a decrease or loss of orgasmic sensation as well.

Pain Following vaginoplasty, individuals may report continued pain with intercourse. This pain is multimodal and can include difficulties with dilation, adequate lubrication, and inability to relax the pelvic floor muscles. The latter may be due not only to disruption of the pelvic floor muscles during surgery, but also to psychosocial factors including anxiety and history of sexual trauma as discussed in the previous sections. Following surgery, 36% of transfeminine individuals were found to have pelvic floor dysfunction including urinary (28%) and fecal incontinence (22%), and severe pelvic pain (28%) [10]. The authors of this study highlighted the utility of pelvic floor physical therapy following gender-affirming vaginoplasty where 69% of participants had resolution of their pelvic floor dysfunction and 89% reported successful dilation at 3 months [10].

Satisfaction

While transfeminine individuals report varying levels of functional disturbances (with or without distress), as noted, this population remains sexually active. The level of sexual satisfaction is related not only to factors surrounding desire and function but also related to where an individual is at in their treatment course. Transfeminine people with fulfilled treatment desire (regardless of the type of treatment received) report high sexual agency, pleasure, and esteem [2]. While this study did not find a difference in satisfaction, they noted the level of satisfaction in this study's population was lower than the general population. However, when looking at factors correlated with sexual satisfaction, unfulfilled treatment was correlated with lower satisfaction, while psychological well-being and body satisfaction were correlated with higher satisfaction.

Future Directions

There remain significant gaps in the literature regarding sexual health, desire, and function in the transfeminine population. Notably is the lack of validated, standardized assessments. Additional stratification by subgroups within this diverse population, such as by treatment an individual has received, additional treatment desired, and current sexual activities and goals, could provide more information. Particular focus may also be placed on the source of pain in this population both during and after intercourse.

Related to pain is the utility of pelvic floor physical therapy both pre- and post-surgery. Given that transfeminine individuals are reporting both pre-treatment and during hormone therapy dyspareunia, and given the noted pelvic floor dysfunction prevalence prior to surgery, a pelvic floor evaluation may be warranted even in those not desiring surgery. Understanding the changes in the pelvic floor during hormone therapy, if any, may also help improve sexual function.

Additionally, there may be utility in continued counseling and mental health resources. Individuals may continue to have feelings of gender dysphoria even after surgery and simply desire additional support as they recover from surgery. Such services could improve sexual health outcomes. Beyond formal counseling and mental health resources, individuals also seek support from the community directly and/or through online networks. Through platforms like Reddit, individuals both seek information and share experiences regarding their surgical experience including changes in sexual function [19]. Such platforms may provide an avenue for physicians to share desired health information regarding sexual function.

Though this chapter focused on sexual function related to genitals, chest feminization surgery can increase overall body satisfaction and impact sexual well-being as well. Ensuring full spectrum, timely, and accessible gender-focused care can help improve overall sexual health and satisfaction in transfeminine individuals.

Conclusion

Transfeminine individuals are sexually active at all stages of their gender affirmation, though the population's desires and goals are heterogenous. Optimizing sexual function requires an interdisciplinary approach but can lead to improvement in the individual's quality of life.

References

1. World Health Organization. Defining sexual health: report of a technical consultation on sexual health, 28–31 January 2002. Geneva: World Health Organization; 2006.
2. Nikkelen SW, Kreukels BP. Sexual experiences in transgender people: the role of desire for gender-confirming interventions, psychological well-being, and body satisfaction. J Sex Marital Ther. 2018;44(4):370–81.
3. Cerwenka S, Nieder TO, Cohen-Kettenis P, De Cuypere G, Haraldsen IRH, Kreukels BP, Richter-Appelt H. Sexual behavior of gender-dysphoric individuals before gender-confirming interventions: a European multicenter study. J Sex Marital Ther. 2014;40(5):457–71.
4. Holmberg M, Arver S, Dhejne C. Supporting sexuality and improving sexual function in transgender persons. Nat Rev Urol. 2019;16(2):121–39.
5. Smith JR, Washington AZ III, Morrison SD, Gottlieb LJ. Assessing patient satisfaction among transgender individuals seeking medical services. Ann Plast Surg. 2018;81(6):725–9.
6. Reisner SL, Poteat T, Keatley J, Cabral M, Mothopeng T, Dunham E, Baral SD, et al. Global health burden and needs of transgender populations: a review. Lancet. 2016;388(10042):412–36.
7. Herbst JH, Jacobs ED, Finlayson TJ, McKleroy VS, Neumann MS, Crepaz N, HIV/AIDS Prevention Research Synthesis Team. Estimating HIV prevalence and risk behaviors of transgender persons in the United States: a systematic review. AIDS Behav. 2008;12(1):1–17.
8. Kerckhof ME, Kreukels BP, Nieder TO, Becker-Hébly I, van de Grift TC, Staphorsius AS, Elaut E, et al. Prevalence of sexual dysfunctions in transgender persons: results from the ENIGI follow-up study. J Sex Med. 2019;16(12):2018–29.
9. Gizewski ER, Krause E, Schlamann M, Happich F, Ladd ME, Forsting M, Senf W. Specific cerebral activation due to visual erotic stimuli in male-to-female transsexuals compared with male and female controls: an fMRI study. J Sex Med. 2009;6(2):440–8.
10. Jiang DD, Gallagher S, Burchill L, Berli J, Dugi D III. Implementation of a pelvic floor physical therapy program for transgender women undergoing gender-affirming vaginoplasty. Obstet Gynecol. 2019;133(5):1003–11.
11. Defreyne J, Elaut E, Kreukels B, Fisher AD, Castellini G, Staphorsius A, T'Sjoen G. Sexual desire changes in transgender individuals upon initiation of hormone treatment: results from the longitudinal European network for the investigation of gender incongruence. J Sex Med. 2020.
12. Ristori J, Cocchetti C, Castellini G, Pierdominici M, Cipriani A, Testi D, et al. Hormonal treatment effect on sexual distress in transgender persons: 2-year follow-up data. J Sex Med. 2020;17(1):142–51.
13. Kronawitter D, Gooren LJ, Zollver H, Oppelt PG, Beckmann MW, Dittrich R, Mueller A. Effects of transdermal testosterone or oral dydrogesterone on hypoactive sexual desire disorder in transsexual women: results of a pilot study. Eur J Endocrinol. 2009;161(2):363.
14. Bettocchi C, Palumbo F, Cormio LUIGI, Ditonno P, Battaglia M, Selvaggi FP. The effects of androgen depletion on human erectile function: a prospective study in male-to-female transsexuals. Int J Impot Res. 2004;16(6):544–6.
15. Hendrix SL, Cochrane BB, Nygaard IE, Handa VL, Barnabei VM, Iglesia C, et al. Effects of estrogen with and without progestin on urinary incontinence. JAMA. 2005;293(8):935–48.
16. Horbach SE, Bouman MB, Smit JM, Özer M, Buncamper ME, Mullender MG. Outcome of vaginoplasty in male-to-female transgenders: a systematic review of surgical techniques. J Sex Med. 2015;12(6):1499–512.
17. Buncamper ME, Honselaar JS, Bouman MB, Özer M, Kreukels BP, Mullender MG. Aesthetic and functional outcomes of neovaginoplasty using penile skin in male-to-female transsexuals. J Sex Med. 2015;12(7):1626–34.
18. Herbenick D, Reece M, Sanders SA, Dodge B, Ghassemi A, Fortenberry JD. Women's vibrator use in sexual partnerships: results from a nationally representative survey in the United States. J Sex Marital Ther. 2010;36(1):49–65.
19. Latack KR, Adidharma W, Moog D, Satterwhite T, Hadj-Moussa M, Morrison SD. Are we preparing patients for gender-affirming surgery? A thematic social media analysis. Plast Reconstruct Surg. 2020;146(4):519e-21e.

Chapter 10
Psychosocial Aspects of Reproduction in Transgender and Non-binary Individuals

Mariam Maksutova and Angela K. Lawson

Introduction

As has been made clear in other chapters in this book, gender identity and the sex assigned to an infant at birth are not equivalent concepts. Gender identity development begins in early childhood and is influenced by a multitude of internal and external factors. In some cases, this process is made more complex and dynamic by nonconformity to societal expectations based on sex assigned at birth (i.e., gender non-conformity), dysphoria (i.e., distress associated with the inconsistency between sex assigned at birth and gender identity), or a combination of both. In transgender and non-binary (TGNB) individuals, the onset of puberty may further exacerbate these feelings and result in gender-related distress [1]. Pathologizing of gender variance by healthcare professionals also starts early. Qualification of presence and severity of gender dysphoria, calculations of the probability of "persistence" in one's gender identity, and numerous psychological evaluations all attempt to identify the bounds of the TGNB experience and, ultimately, determine when and for whom medical intervention is appropriate [2–4].

M. Maksutova
University of Michigan Medical School, Ann Arbor, MI, USA
e-mail: mmaksut@med.umich.edu

A. K. Lawson (✉)
Department of Obstetrics & Gynecology, Northwestern University, Chicago, IL, USA
e-mail: alawson@nm.org

© The Author(s), under exclusive license to Springer Nature Switzerland AG 2023
M. B. Moravek, G. de Haan (eds.), *Reproduction in Transgender and Nonbinary Individuals*, https://doi.org/10.1007/978-3-031-14933-7_10

Barriers to Medical Care

Likely due to community activism and an increase in media visibility, awareness of TGNB-specific healthcare needs has increased over the last decade. Development of Endocrine Society and World Professional Association for Transgender Health (WPATH) clinical practice guidelines and updates to the Diagnostic and Statistical Manual of Mental Disorders (DSM-5) have improved access to, and quality of, care for some. For example, the DSM-IV diagnostic category of Gender Identity Disorder (which appeared to suggest that the individual's incongruent beliefs between their sex assigned at birth and their gender identity was pathologic) has been replaced in the DSM-5 with a new category of Gender Dysphoria and focuses on the distress one may experience as a result of this incongruence, rather than the incongruence itself. Development of more pediatric multidisciplinary gender clinics and rising numbers of TGNB youth presenting for gender services also demonstrate movement in a more inclusive, culturally competent direction [3, 5].

Despite this encouraging trajectory, many barriers to medical care, including reproductive care, persist for TGNB individuals. These include systemic barriers of varying degrees, from lack of insurance coverage for gender-affirming services, lack of provider training, misidentification on medical ID bracelets, lack of proper accommodations (e.g., bathrooms), and cisgender/binary design of the Electronic Medical Record and patient healthcare forms. On an interpersonal level, social stigma, cultural prejudice, harassment, and discrimination are still common within healthcare facilities and in the public sector. Humiliating treatment, insensitivity, discrimination, name-calling, and even violence perpetrated by healthcare providers against TGNB individuals is well chronicled [6–8]. These experiences themselves, along with the ambient environment of collective trauma resulting from their prevalence within the TGNB community, lead to delay and avoidance of medical care, unsupervised hormone use, increased risk of non-adherence to medical advice, and psychological distress. For example, a 2015 national survey of 27,715 transgender adults found that, of 12,037 individuals using hormones, 9% were using nonprescription hormones [9]. Furthermore, in a recent study of 433 transgender people in Ontario, Canada, one in five reported avoiding the emergency department due to fear of transphobia and discrimination [10].

In addition to being a barrier to competent medical care, transphobia is a significant psychological stressor for TGNB individuals. TGNB people experience significantly higher rates of harassment, victimization, and violence compared to their cisgender peers [11]. The dysphoria experienced by many TGNB individuals further adds to the psychological burden of these individuals [12]. Of course, neither dysphoria nor transphobia are prerequisites for TGNB identity, but both are common components of many narratives. As a result of the many real barriers and stressors faced by TGNB individuals, this population is at a vastly increased risk for anxiety/depression, suicidality, self-injury, lower academic performance, substance use, family conflict, and violence. A 2017 study by Nahata et al. found that of 78 medical records of individuals diagnosed with gender dysphoria, 92% were diagnosed with depression, anxiety, post-traumatic stress disorder, eating disorders, autism spectrum disorder, bipolar disorder, or a combination of these conditions [13]. Another study found that TGNB individuals have a 44% risk of developing depression and a 33% risk of developing anxiety. Between 41% and 60% of transgender individuals have attempted suicide, a stark contrast to the 2–4.6% among the general population [2, 12]. However, it is important to note that this increase in risk is not inherent to TGNB identity and is more strongly associated with the challenges that TGNB individuals face in modern society. This is well supported by findings that gender-affirming care and gender-affirming behavior decrease the risk of mental health conditions to that of general population averages [2].

Barriers to Competent Reproductive Care

Although the availability of gender-affirming care appears to be increasing, TGNB individuals still may not receive needed counseling regarding their future reproductive needs or may experience barriers to receipt of fertility care which may also result in psychological distress. For example, some TGNB people choose to undergo medical transition to affirm their gender identity. Medical transition is an umbrella term and can include Gender-Affirming Hormone (GAH) therapy (e.g., estrogen, testosterone, and endogenous hormone blockers) and Gender-Affirming Surgery (GAS) (e.g., mastectomy, phalloplasty, vaginoplasty, and gonadectomy). Not all TGNB people pursue medical transition and this does not delegitimize an individual's TGNB identity. For those who have the means and desire to engage with such services, medical transition has been shown to have an overwhelmingly positive effect on quality of life and mental health. Consistently, studies have found that GAH and GAS contribute to increased self-esteem, family support, and quality of life and interpersonal relationships, while reducing concerns about gender-related discrimination and violence [14–18].

However, long-standing exposure to testosterone in transmasculine individuals and estrogen in transfeminine individuals has been shown to *potentially* negatively affect oocyte production and spermatogenesis [19], respectively, and gonadectomy results in sterilization. Any resulting impairment of reproductive ability by these medical interventions has often been accepted as the "price to pay" for gender-affirming treatment. Loss of fertility has been previously described as a logical and therapeutic part of the "transition process" essential for fully breaking with the gender incorrectly assigned at birth [20, 21]. In the last decade, mandatory sterilization prior to transition has been banned in a number of countries, including Sweden (2013), France (2016), and Belgium (2017). In others, such as Greece, Japan, Russia, Switzerland, and Turkey, the practice remains an active standard of care [20].

In addition to the emotional toll of lost biological fertility, TGNB individuals often face transphobic stereotypes that they are incompetent parents or, worse yet, create a detrimental environment for growing children. Although there is no evidence that having a transgender parent affects a child's gender identity development

[22], overt transphobia, and unconscious bias, as well as the need to battle these, has fueled numerous investigations into whether TGNB people could ever be "good" parents [21, 23, 24]. Incorrect and unfounded assumptions about the negative influence of parents' TGNB identities on their children's gender identity and sexual orientation are a frustrating and common barrier to family building for this population due to fear and/or presence of discrimination [25]. For example, in a study describing the experiences of transgender men around pregnancy, several respondents described social services threatening or attempting to remove their children from their care, sometimes before the birth and in one case lasting years, afterward [26]. Together, the accepted expectation of sacrificing fertility for gender affirmation and the misconception that TGNB people are poor parents has led many to believe that transness and reproduction are inherently at odds. Though the physiological effects of gender-affirming hormones and surgeries are not a novel discovery, it has taken until 2001 for a paragraph recommending discussion of fertility preservation (FP) before hormone initiation to be added to the WPATH standards of care [19, 25].

Parenthood Desires

Despite the increased stigma historically surrounding LGBTQ conception, pregnancy, and childrearing, and like many cisgender adults, many TGNB adults long to be parents. A 2002 questionnaire of transgender women ($n = 121$) showed that 77% of those asked thought that fertility preservation (FP) was important to discuss and should have been offered by their healthcare provider. The same study found that for transfeminine individuals, "regret at not being able to become pregnant themselves" was a recurring theme and that 67% of these individuals under age 40 would have considered sperm freezing, or chosen to do so, had it been offered prior to hormone initiation [27]. Similarly, a survey of transgender men ($n = 50$) showed that more than half had a desire to have genetically related children, and 37.5% would have cryopreserved oocytes if it had been possible at the time [22]. More recently, a survey found that 47% of transgender respondents wished to have a child to whom they are genetically related [28]. Of note, transgender people with children, biological, or otherwise, scored substantially higher on mental health and vitality scores than those without children [22], demonstrating that the inability to have biologic children (e.g., forced sterilization) is not likely to be therapeutic after all.

The psychological desire to parent is strong among many TGNB adults. Among TGNB adolescents, statistics related to FP look markedly different. At one specialty clinic ($n = 72$), 97% of young people with documented fertility counseling declined to consider further gamete preserving interventions [19]. In this cohort, commonly cited reasons included plans to adopt, no desire to have children, cost, discomfort with procedures, and concerns about delaying hormone treatment. A different study of 105 adolescents who received initial fertility counseling documented only 12.4% as pursuing a formal FP consultation and less than 5% cryopreserving gametes [29].

At first, it may be easy to attribute this discrepancy between reported desires in adolescents and adults to youths having difficulty envisioning and making decisions about future family building. However, in similarly aged individuals requiring FP for chronic illness (cancer, lupus, etc.), concern about the loss of fertility and utilization of gamete preserving services is notably higher [19, 30].

Although the reason for the difference in FP between TGNB youth and youth with medical illnesses has not yet been fully elucidated TGNB youth must often contend with additional layers of stigma, societal expectations, and harassment compared to their cisgender peers [2, 12, 13]. Additionally, FP for an adolescent with a chronic illness may be covered by insurance, while TGNB individuals are likely to have to fight harder for coverage at every step and are nearly certain to be denied or have only partial coverage for services that are prohibitively expensive for most people [9]. Gamete preservation among TGNB youth is often presented as an extra step to "opt-in" whereas it is seen as an expected part of treatment for young patients with cancer or other diseases which require gonadotoxic interventions [31]. Additionally, parental involvement may look different for these two groups. While a great majority of parents of children with a new cancer diagnosis reported their child's fertility being a priority [32], only half of the surveyed parents of TGNB youth reported wanting to learn about and wanting their children to consider FP. Less than one-third of parents of TGNB youth reported they wanted their children to undergo FP [33]. In a study of transgender youth asked about their relationships with their parents ($n = 55$), participants reported that 54% of their mothers and 63% of their fathers initially reacted negatively to their gender identity, and 50% of the mothers and 44% of their fathers still felt negatively at the time of the interviews, an average of 3 years later [34]. When controlled for demographic variables, parental support is significantly associated with higher life satisfaction, lower perceived burden, and fewer depressive symptoms [35]. This is the very support that TGNB youth are at a much higher risk of not receiving, and the lack or reduction of parental support may be responsible for a sense of hopelessness regarding the potential for adult happiness and family satisfaction, which makes future childrearing more challenging to imagine for TGNB youth. It may also result in a failure of parents of TGNB youth to adequately value or advocate for their children's reproductive needs [33].

Interestingly, when asked, many TGNB adolescents expressed a greater interest in pursuing adoption than biological parenthood [19, 36]. In one survey of TGNB youth, 70.5% of 156 respondents were interested in adoption compared to 35.9% interested in biological parenthood [36]. Research in this area is limited, but this large preference toward adoption may be, at least in part, due to unrealistic expectations about the process. While adoption is less physically invasive and therefore less likely to trigger feelings of gender dysphoria than FP, it is also likely to be experienced as an emotional roller coaster as it is not easy, cheap, or free from discrimination. The wait to adopt a healthy infant in the United States often lasts several years and LGBTQ+ prospective parents seeking to adopt face a host of unique legal challenges [37] as well as opening themselves up to transphobia and stigma. In addition to interpersonal discrimination, "religious freedom" laws, currently in place in ten states, permit systemic discrimination against LGBTQ+ adoptive and foster parents on the basis of an organization's religious beliefs [38].

Considering this context, it is clear that a great deal of planning and perseverance through emotional stressors may be necessary for TGNB people working to grow their families. In a survey of 291 TGNB parents asked to identify their pathway to parenthood, 60% reported that they were co-biological parents with a partner, 23% reported that their partner was a biological parent but they were not, 13% reported that they were a biological parent without a co-biological parent partner, and 5% reported being adoptive or foster parents [39]. In those desiring a genetic relationship to their child, biological parenthood may be possible with or without medical intervention. Both paths come with their own unique sets of challenges, and the biological capabilities and preferences of the aspiring parent(s) must be taken into account. There are multiple possible combinations of gametes, reproductive organs, and desires that inform decision-making related to family building [25]. In a partnership without both viable sperm and oocytes, conversations about which parent will be biologically related to the child are necessary. Often, conception may require a third-party, in the form of a sperm or oocyte donor or surrogate, and thus the involvement of the legal system (e.g., regarding parenting rights, third-party rights, and financial compensation), which may create emotional complications within family dynamics (e.g., when a nongenetic parent feels unequal in family building roles). Legal considerations for family building are further explored in Chap. 11.

Gamete cryopreservation, fertilization, and implantation are time and resource (e.g., financial and psychological) consuming. It can be difficult, even impossible, to access these expensive and invasive options. The number of required decisions (e.g., which partner's gametes to use, which donor to select), potential loss of genetic connections, and the need for consideration of disclosure of third-party reproduction to children may pose psychological barriers to treatment [21, 25, 28, 40]. For TGNB individuals who pursue family building, fertility clinics, sperm banks, egg donor and gestational carrier agencies, and birth wards are often designed to cater to a binary cisgender clientele among whom gender roles are firmly established. Such environments, as well as genital examinations and the physical changes associated with discontinuation of hormone treatment or pregnancy for transmasculine patients who either desire to carry or are unable to afford gestational surrogacy fees may trigger tremendous gender incongruence and dysphoria [41]. For example, one transgender man described his experience of stopping hormones to begin FP as *"Ceasing to take testosterone so that the [bleeding] would reappear was one of the hardest things. [GA: How has it been?] It has been very tough. It was tough mentally to discontinue. [...] It affects everything; I could feel how I smelled differently when I didn't use testosterone. [...] Then I noticed it mentally also. I was back in the more ... What to say? ... varying hormone cycle ... that I don't really appreciate"* [41].

In addition to internal emotional struggles such as dysphoria and realistic fears of discrimination and/or hostility while undergoing fertility treatment, transphobia does not end where prenatal care starts. One qualitative study describes that most participants reported having to choose between concealing their identity and other medically relevant information in order to receive compassionate care or disclosing their identity and risking being subjected to invasive procedures and inappropriate questions that felt objectifying [26].

Family planning can be an emotionally complex experience for anyone who engages in it, regardless of gender identity, gender expression, sexual orientation, or sex assigned at birth. However, TGNB individuals desiring biological offspring face additional emotional hurdles. Infertility alone can lead to self-blame, anger, and sadness. Dysphoria and acute mental distress when attempting to conceive (changes to physical appearance, the onset of menses, distress with masturbation, genital exams, etc.) can be severe. In pregnancy, there can be both an emotional toll on an individual for whom the act is incongruent with their gender as well as for couples and individuals who must reconcile the involvement of third-party reproductive assistance. Many describe these experiences as being incredibly isolating. For example, one transgender man pursuing pregnancy stated: *"I looked at it as something to endure to have a child."* [42] TGNB parents may also receive less support if they experience pregnancy loss and bereavement if their family building experience is difficult for friends and family to understand. If all goes to plan and their experience results in a healthy child, trans parents do not always have the legal protections of their cis counterparts. For example, in the case of *Cisek v. Cisek*, a court terminated the visitation rights of a transgender parent, holding that there was a risk of both mental and "social harm" to the children [43]. Additionally, TGNB individuals likely fear and often endure judgment and discrimination from those who do not believe that TGNB people should be allowed to be parents in the first place.

Problems with and Solutions to the Current Medical System

As previously described, the modern medical system has historically caused psychological and physical harm to the TGNB community (e.g., discrimination and sterilization). TGNB individuals have and continue to face additional challenges relative to their cisgender counterparts when it comes to having both their reproductive and general healthcare needs met. Overall, the obstacles TGNB people face in accessing competent and compassionate healthcare have been described as falling into three distinct categories: estrangement, expectations, and eviction [44]. "Estrangement" encompasses barriers to initiating care that arise due to lack of knowledge among providers. It encompasses everything from "Trans Broken Arm Syndrome" (i.e., healthcare providers' assumption that all medical issues, from disordered mental health to broken bones, are a result of a patient's TGNB identity) to the burden often put on TGNB individuals to educate providers about their bodies. "Expectations" refers to the cis/hetero-normative assumptions providers often make about TGNB patients. This includes assumptions about gender, sexual orientation, relationship status, and transition goals, all of which vary among TGNB people just as they do among cisgender people. Non-binary and gender fluid individuals, who often do not fit neatly into traditional transgender narratives, must additionally contend with the linear expectations of transgender care and assumptions about desired physiological and social trajectory. Finally, "Eviction," or feelings of abandonment by providers after certain healthcare milestones had been met, often leads to oversight of general wellness and health needs unrelated to TGNB identity such as lack of trans-inclusive counseling for postpartum depression. These healthcare failures combine with others (personal, social, financial) to restrict access to care for TGNB patients and worsen the emotional burden faced by TGNB people receiving medical care.

Before beginning a conversation about improving trans-competence, support, and access in our hospitals and clinics, it is important to acknowledge that for as long as there have been barriers, there have been TGNB people circumnavigating them. For most, seeking competent care is an active decision. "After enduring discrimination and insensitive treatment, most described a point in time in which they decided to seek healthcare that met their unique needs as [transgender individuals] rather than follow a generic health care path." [45] Because training in TGNB-specific care and provider exposure to TGNB patients is sorely lacking [3, 46], patients must often do a great deal of research independently, before establishing care with a provider. For example, *"But so I told her [the doctor] that I had done my due diligence, that I had spent 8 years researching medical transition, social transition, legal aspects of transition, that I knew what I was getting into, that I was quite well informed."* Familiarity with the healthcare system can be key to maneuver around it, *"The loophole that my doctor uses for every single [transgender] patient is he'll just bill the insurance or he'll write it off as hormone imbalance instead of . . . transgender."* Additional effort to receive competent care is also required, such as traveling long distances to see competent providers, continually working on relationships to ensure that providers are aware of needs and concerns, and "playing the long game" by putting off necessary care. For example, *"I waited because I knew I was transgender. I wanted a hysterectomy but I knew that my insurance would not cover it. .... I had an abnormal Pap smear prior to me getting cervical cancer. ... I waited and I did not go back in for any kind of Pap smear. I did not go back in for any pelvic exams, I waited 6 years until .... it was just something that came over my body that I knew that okay, I pushed it far enough, I should go in, and I did and I was just at that point where [it] was CIN3 (e.g., cervical intraepithelial neoplasia).... But so I knew and since it had been far enough, my insurance covered my hysterectomy."* [45].

In order to work toward restoring TGNB people's faith in and reduce distress associated with the healthcare system, training regarding this population's needs is essential for healthcare providers and clinic staff. This is true of reproductive needs as well as TGNB health more broadly. More knowledgeable, confident providers will, in turn, be better equipped to counsel patients. "Although TGNB family creation role models and information are increasing, it is critical for TGNB people to have easy access to accurate, empowering information" from their healthcare providers "that can guide their thinking and inform their choices in family creation." [21].

Furthermore, patients undergoing potentially gonadotoxic treatment should receive FP counseling. Similar to the American Society for Reproductive Medicine recommendations for patients seeking FP prior to gonadotoxic treatment and patients utilizing third-party preproduction [31], consultation with a mental health professional who specializes in reproductive medicine is warranted with the FP referral and at family building initiation. Anticipatory guidance from a mental health provider should address mood, presence or absence of support systems, need for third-party assistance, psychoeducation regarding treatment, informed decision-making and decision regret, realistic treatment expectations, body dysphoria, concerns about treatment as a TGNB individual and coping strategies. Because TGNB people have historically had a complex relationship with mental health providers (e.g., mandatory mental health assessments prior to GAH initiation or GAS clearance, gatekeeping, having one's identity attributed to a DSM diagnosis, and toxic and abusive nature of "transgender conversion" therapy) providers must proceed with care and should have specialty training in working with TGNB patient populations. FP for TGNB individuals as part of medical transition decision-making is integral to ensuring patients are well-informed and prepared to make complex decisions about their health and their future. However, emphasis must be placed on support rather than screening, and such counseling must be readily available, affordable, and an option for all patients.

It is also the responsibility of healthcare professionals to make offices, clinics, and hospital rooms affirming and safe spaces for TGNB patients. Staples of working toward this goal include provision of gender neutral materials and forms, inclusive verbal communication, and familiarity with relevant literature and legal information. Following the patient's cues when discussing physiology, experiences, and sensitive subjects, and apologizing when mistakes are made, is paramount. For patients who use a name that differs from the one given at birth, affirmation of chosen name should be the standard of care, as it is well documented to reduce mental health risks such as depression, suicidal ideation, and suicidal behavior. Likewise, asking for and consistently using correct pronouns can be a lifesaving measure [47, 48]. Appropriate names and pronouns (i.e., those identified as such by the individual they refer to) should be used even when the patient is not present in order to engage in the respectful care of TGNB individuals.

Conclusions

Overall, growing one's family as a TGNB individual is often an emotionally involved and complex journey. TGNB youth must grow up in a world that is not designed with them in mind. A world in which, for them, discrimination, hostility, and rejection often play a prominent role. Upon entering adulthood, TGNB adults must continue to overcome psychological, interpersonal, and systemic barriers to access quality healthcare. As these individuals plan and grow families, there is a tremendous risk they will be exposed to further harm in fertility clinics, ObGyn clinics, and birth wards. As healthcare professionals, we can, and we must, do better. This starts with awareness of the context within which these patients present. Of course, just like cisgender people, TGNB people come from a variety of backgrounds and experiences, and there is no one-size-fits-all way of providing competent care. However, most missteps can be avoided by using gender neutral terms for body parts and procedures, using correct names and pronouns, providing a welcoming clinic environment for all patients, and not reducing the identity of a diverse community to a pathology.

References

1. de Vries AL, McGuire JK, Steensma TD, Wagenaar EC, Doreleijers TA, Cohen-Kettenis PT. Young adult psychological outcome after puberty suppression and gender reassignment. Pediatrics. 2014;134(4):696–704.
2. Guss C, Shumer D, Katz-Wise SL. Transgender and gender nonconforming adolescent care: psychosocial and medical considerations. Curr Opin Pediatr. 2015;27(4):421–6.
3. Vance SR Jr, Ehrensaft D, Rosenthal SM. Psychological and medical care of gender nonconforming youth. Pediatrics. 2014;134(6):1184–92.
4. Steensma TD, Biemond R, de Boer F, Cohen-Kettenis PT. Desisting and persisting gender dysphoria after childhood: a qualitative follow-up study. Clin Child Psychol Psychiatry. 2011;16(4):499–516.
5. Roberts TK, Fantz CR. Barriers to quality health care for the transgender population. Clin Biochem. 2014;47(10–11):983–7.
6. Shires DA, Jaffee K. Factors associated with health care discrimination experiences among a national sample of female-to-male transgender individuals. Health Soc Work. 2015;40(2):134–41.
7. Shaffer N. Transgender patients: implications for emergency department policy and practice. J Emerg Nurs. 2005;31(4):405–7.
8. James SE, Herman JL, Rankin S, Keisling M, Mottet L, Anafi M. The report of the 2015 U.S. transgender survey. Washington, DC: National Center for Transgender Equality; 2016.
9. Stroumsa D, Crissman HP, Dalton VK, Kolenic G, Richardson CR. Insurance coverage and use of hormones among transgender respondents to a National Survey. Ann Fam Med. 2020;18(6):528–34.
10. Bauer GR, Scheim AI, Deutsch MB, Massarella C. Reported emergency department avoidance, use, and experiences of transgender persons in Ontario, Canada: results from a respondent-driven sampling survey. Ann Emerg Med. 2014;63(6):713–20. e711
11. Langenderfer-Magruder L, Walls NE, Kattari SK, Whitfield DL, Ramos D. Sexual victimization and subsequent police reporting by gender identity among lesbian, gay, bisexual, transgender, and queer adults. Violence Vict. 2016;31(2):320–31.
12. Olson J, Schrager SM, Belzer M, Simons LK, Clark LF. Baseline physiologic and psychosocial characteristics of transgender youth seeking Care for Gender Dysphoria. J Adolesc Health. 2015;57(4):374–80.
13. Nahata L, Quinn GP, Caltabellotta NM, Tishelman AC. Mental health concerns and insurance denials among transgender adolescents. LGBT Health. 2017;4(3):188–93.
14. Gorin-Lazard A, Baumstarck K, Boyer L, et al. Hormonal therapy is associated with better self-esteem, mood, and quality of life in transsexuals. J Nerv Ment Dis. 2013;201(11):996–1000.
15. Branstrom R, Pachankis JE. Reduction in mental health treatment utilization among transgender individuals after gender-affirming surgeries: a Total population study. Am J Psychiatry. 2020;177(8):727–34.
16. Ozata Yildizhan B, Yuksel S, Avayu M, Noyan H, Yildizhan E. Effects of gender reassignment on quality of life and mental health in people with gender dysphoria. Turk Psikiyatri Derg. 2018;29(1):11–21.

17. Wernick JA, Busa S, Matouk K, Nicholson J, Janssen A. A systematic review of the psychological benefits of gender-affirming surgery. Urol Clin North Am. 2019;46(4):475–86.
18. Schmidt L, Levine R. Psychological outcomes and reproductive issues among gender dysphoric individuals. Endocrinol Metab Clin N Am. 2015;44(4):773–85.
19. Nahata L, Tishelman AC, Caltabellotta NM, Quinn GP. Low fertility preservation utilization among transgender youth. J Adolesc Health. 2017;61(1):40–4.
20. De Sutter P. The desire to have children and the preservation of fertility in transsexual women: a survey. Int J Transgend. 2002;6:215–21.
21. Dickey LM, Ducheny KM, Ehrbar RD. Family creation options for transgender and gender nonconforming people. Psychol Sex Orientat Gend Divers. 2016;3:173–9.
22. Wierckx K, Van Caenegem E, Pennings G, et al. Reproductive wish in transsexual men. Hum Reprod. 2012;27(2):483–7.
23. Bos HM, Knox JR, van Rijn-van GL, Gartrell NK. Same-sex and different-sex parent households and child health outcomes: findings from the National Survey of Children's Health. J Dev Behav Pediatr. 2016;37(3):179–87.
24. White T, Ettner R. Adaptation and adjustment in children of transsexual parents. Eur Child Adolesc Psychiatry. 2007;16(4):215–21.
25. T'Sjoen G, Van Caenegem E, Wierckx K. Transgenderism and reproduction. Curr Opin Endocrinol Diabetes Obes. 2013;20(6):575–9.
26. Hoffkling A, Obedin-Maliver J, Sevelius J. From erasure to opportunity: a qualitative study of the experiences of transgender men around pregnancy and recommendations for providers. BMC Pregnancy Childbirth. 2017;17(Suppl 2):332.
27. De Sutter P, Kira K, Verschoor A, Hotimsky A. The desire to have children and the preservation of fertility in transsexual women: a survey. Int J Transgend. 2002;6(3):215–21.
28. Tornello SL, Bos H. Parenting intentions among transgender individuals. Lgbt Health. 2017;4(2):115–20.
29. Chen D, Simons L, Johnson EK, Lockart BA, Finlayson C. Fertility preservation for transgender adolescents. J Adolesc Health. 2017;61(1):120–3.
30. Strang JF, Jarin J, Call D, et al. Transgender youth fertility attitudes questionnaire: measure development in nonautistic and autistic transgender youth and their parents. J Adolesc Health. 2018;62(2):128–35.
31. Practice Committee of the American Society for Reproductive Medicine. Fertility preservation in patients undergoing gonadotoxic therapy or gonadectomy: a committee opinion. Fertil Steril. 2019;112:1022–33.
32. Oosterhuis BE, Goodwin T, Kiernan M, Hudson MM, Dahl GV. Concerns about infertility risks among pediatric oncology patients and their parents. Pediatr Blood Cancer. 2008;50:85–9.
33. Nahata L, Curci MB, Quinn GP. Exploring fertility preservation intentions among transgender youth. J Adolesc Health. 2018;62(2):123–5.
34. Grossman AH, D'Augelli AR, Howell TJ, Hubbard S. Parent' reactions to transgender Youth' gender nonconforming expression and identity. J Gay Lesbian Social Serv. 2008;18:3–16.
35. Simons L, Schrager SM, Clark LF, Belzer M, Olson J. Parental support and mental health among transgender adolescents. J Adolesc Health. 2013;53(6):791–3.
36. Chen D, Matson M, Macapagal K, et al. Attitudes toward fertility and reproductive health among transgender and gender-nonconforming adolescents. J Adolesc Health. 2018;63(1):62–8.
37. Farr RH, Goldberg AE. Sexual orientation, gender identity, and adoption law. Fam Court Rev. 2018;56:374–83.
38. Movement Advancement Project. Non-discrimination laws. www.lgbtmap.org/equality-maps/non_discrimination_laws. Accessed February 2, 2020.
39. Tornello SL, Riskind RG, Babic A. Transgender and gender non-binary parents' pathways to parenthood. Psychol Sex Orientat Gend Divers. 2019;6:232–41.
40. De Roo C, Tilleman K, T'Sjoen G, De Sutter P. Fertility options in transgender people. Int Rev Psychiatry. 2016;28(1):112–9.

41. Armuand G, Dhejne C, Olofsson JI, Rodriguez-Wallberg KA. Transgender men's experiences of fertility preservation: a qualitative study. Hum Reprod. 2017;32(2):383–90.
42. Light AD, Obedin-Maliver J, Sevelius JM, Kerns JL. Transgender men who experienced pregnancy after female-to-male gender transitioning. Obstet Gynecol. 2014;124(6):1120–7.
43. Cooper L. Protecting the rights of transgender parents and their children: a guide for parents and lawyers. New York, NY: Americal Civil Liberties Union; 2013.
44. Lindroth M. 'Competent persons who can treat you with competence, as simple as that'—an interview study with transgender people on their experiences of meeting health care professionals. J Clin Nurs. 2016;25(23–24):3511–21.
45. Roller CG, Sedlak C, Draucker CB. Navigating the system: how transgender individuals engage in health care services. J Nurs Scholarsh. 2015;47(5):417–24.
46. Vance SR Jr, Halpern-Felsher BL, Rosenthal SM. Health care providers' comfort with and barriers to care of transgender youth. J Adolesc Health. 2015;56(2):251–3.
47. Olson KR, Durwood L, DeMeules M, McLaughlin KA. Mental health of transgender children who are supported in their identities. Pediatrics. 2016;137(3):e20153223.
48. Russell ST, Pollitt AM, Li G, Grossman AH. Chosen name use is linked to reduced depressive symptoms, suicidal ideation, and suicidal behavior among transgender youth. J Adolesc Health. 2018;

Chapter 11
Legal Considerations

Will Halm, Eliseo Arebalos, Catherine B. McGowan, Rachael J. Bailey, and Malina Simard-Halm

The paths to fertility preservation and family creation for transgender and non-binary (TGNB) individuals may involve a fair amount of legal and logistical complexity depending on the circumstances of the involved parties. This is especially true when it comes to the law. TGNB individuals must often navigate a complex and rigid legal system that was not designed to accommodate their identities. This presents unique legal hurdles that often require these communities to serve as self-advocates—and occasionally legal pioneers.

In this chapter, we will guide the reader through some of the more frequent legal hurdles that TGNB individuals may encounter as they move forward on their paths to fertility preservation and family creation. We will begin by examining existing legislation impacting these groups, followed by the impact of legal name changes and birth certificate amendments, and conclude by discussing the Patient Protection and Affordable Care Act of 2010 (the "ACA," also known as Obamacare),[1] as well as a few nuances of health care insurance.

---

[1] PATIENT PROTECTION AND AFFORDABLE CARE ACT, PL 111–148, March 23, 2010, 124 Stat 119.

W. Halm (✉) · E. Arebalos · C. B. McGowan · R. J. Bailey · M. Simard-Halm
International Reproductive Law Group Inc., Los Angeles, CA, USA
e-mail: will@irlawgroup.com; eliseo@irlawgroup.com; catherine@irlawgroup.com; rachael@irlawgroup.com; malina@irlawgroup.com

© The Author(s), under exclusive license to Springer Nature
Switzerland AG 2023
M. B. Moravek, G. de Haan (eds.), *Reproduction in Transgender and Nonbinary Individuals*, https://doi.org/10.1007/978-3-031-14933-7_11

Legislation

In its ideal form, legislation represents the will of the people and reflects accepted social norms. Lawmaking may seek to right past wrongs to ensure that future generations do not suffer the same inequities as their predecessors. Furthermore, enacted legislation often strives to give legal recognition to a previously silenced demographic or neglected subject matter that affects the welfare of the nation. When legislation fails to protect the special interests of marginalized groups or contains ambiguity, it creates legal risks and uncertainty for that community. This has long been the case for TGNB individuals seeking fertility preservation treatment and those desiring to create a family who are in need of fertility assistance. We address some of the legal complexities associated with fertility preservation and establishing parentage experienced by many TGNB communities below.

(a) **Fertility Preservation**. There is no federal law requiring insurers to cover fertility preservation generally for TGNB individuals. Fertility workups, by contrast, are generally covered by insurers and available to all those insured,[2] including TGNB individuals.

Though there is no federal legislation requiring insurers to cover fertility preservation, ten states, including California, Connecticut, Delaware, Illinois, Maryland, New Hampshire, New Jersey, New York, and Rhode Island passed legislation requiring fully insured plans[3] to include fertility preservation benefits. While an important step, it is unclear whether these expanded benefits are equally available to TGNB individuals.

For example, California's law requires that fertility preservation benefits be available for infertility "…caused directly or indirectly by surgery, chemotherapy, radiation, or other medical treatment."[4] The last category "other medical treatment" is undefined in California's statute. While California's law identifies standard fertility preservation services as "a basic health care service," the statute's ambiguous language leaves it to insurers to determine whether the fertility preservation benefit extends to TGNB individuals. Thus far, the only insurer in California to affirmatively state that they interpret California's statute to apply to TGNB individuals is Kaiser Permanente.[5]

(b) **Establishing Parentage**. Before embarking on the journey to family creation, it is critical for TGNB individuals to create a plan for establishing their parentage of the child/ren under the law if the creation of their family will involve third-party reproduction, for example, gestational carriers, or donated genetic material. Similar to the lack of legislation relating to fertility preservation for

---

[2] Insurers will typically not cover fertility workups for minors (i.e., under 18 years).

[3] As distinguished from fully insured plans, self-insured or self-funded insurance plans are exempt from state law.

[4] Cal. Health & Safety Code, Section 1374.551.

[5] https://thrive.kaiserpermanente.org/care-near-you/northern-california/eastbay/departments/transgender-care/fertility-preservation/

11 Legal Considerations

TGNB individuals, express legislation providing for and protecting the ability of TGNB couples to create a family if they are unable to do so using their own anatomy and genetic material is non-existent, both at the federal and at the state levels. For TGNB married couples, this may require that they resort to other means to establish or confirm the non-delivering parent's parental rights.[6] This may include relying on marriage, donor insemination statutes, or other agreements to establish parentage under the law.

(i) *Marital Presumption.* One method of establishing the non-delivering parent's parental rights may be through the legal standard of marital presumption. Marital presumption holds that the non-delivering parent is presumed to be the parent of a child born or conceived during the marriage. In that case, both the spouse who gives birth to the child (i.e., the delivering parent) and the other spouse (i.e., the non-delivering parent) will be deemed by default to be equal parents and their names will be reflected as parents on the child's birth certificate. In short, it is the couple's marital status, and not biology, that establishes the non-delivering parent's parental rights.[7]

(ii) *Donor Insemination Statutes.* A second potential method of establishing parentage may be through a state's donor insemination statute. Here, one member of a married couple will undergo artificial insemination using donor sperm.[8, 9] The donor insemination statute may require the insemination to be performed by a licensed physician (i.e., no home inseminations). If a child results from the insemination procedure(s), then the "husband" is the father of the child born to his "wife" through donor insemination. Husband and wife are placed in quotation marks in the preceding sentence as many states have yet to update their statutes to replace husband and wife with gender-neutral terms. As a result, some states may strictly interpret terms such as "woman," "wife," "man," or "husband," depriving the non-delivering parent who does not meet the strict definition of these terms of any parental rights to the child. In that case, the non-delivering parent

---

[6] In the following paragraphs, we will focus on the establishment of parental rights of married couples. A single person who delivers a child is automatically presumed to be a parent to the resulting child. Notwithstanding the information provided in this section, couples seeking to create a family should consult with an attorney who can advise as to the best course of action.

[7] For couples working with a gestational carrier (also known as a surrogate), parentage for both individuals can be established via a surrogacy agreement and/or a declaratory parentage judgment.

[8] To clarify, donor sperm in this instance is sperm from a third-party donor (i.e., not from the other spouse).

[9] It should be noted that a spouse whose sperm is used to artificially inseminate their partner should not sign a form indicating they are waiving parental rights; if anything, the spouse whose sperm will be used should sign a consent form or an acknowledgment indicating they fully intend on being a parent to the child.

would resort to establishing their parental rights by means of a parentage judgment or adoption.[10]

(iii) *Agreement or Memorandum of Intent to Parent.* As may be evident by this point, a certain amount of planning may be indicated prior to TGNB prospective parents beginning the path to family creation. It is advisable that involved parties, prior to beginning their path to family creation, document in writing their understanding of intent and desire to be legal parents to any resulting child. It would also be prudent for the document to note that the non-delivering parent should not be deprived of parentage rights simply because there is no law(s) specifically allowing for those rights to be granted. While these types of memorandums or agreements may not be legally enforceable, they do provide a court with a written account of the involved parties' intentions prior to family creation. These types of memorandums or agreements could be instrumental in future custody disputes, as they may provide the court with a basis for granting a non-delivering parent visitation rights or custody.

Modifications to State and Federal Identification

TGNB individuals may undergo legal name changes, birth certificate amendments, and modifications to other forms of state and federal identification.[11] As with fertility preservation and family creation, careful thought and planning should be given before initiating a change or amendment to identification. The amendment process and timing can be critical; initiating a change at an inopportune time may create additional hurdles for these individuals.

This section identifies some of the potential hurdles for TGNB individuals when one or more changes or amendments to identification remain incomplete. The potential impact this may have on their path to fertility preservation, family creation, or life, generally, is also discussed.

---

[10] Even in instances where the marital presumption or a donor insemination statute may be invoked, many attorneys would still recommend that the non-gestational parent adopt the child given the lack of precedent upholding the rights of nonbiological TGNB parents via either the marital presumption or a donor insemination statute.

[11] The National Center for Transgender Equality provides resources and checklists on their website detailing the various state and federal processes to amend identification, as well as suggestions as to the order in which the changes should be made. See https://transequality.org/documents

11 Legal Considerations

The Challenges of Inconsistent Legal Identification

TGNB individuals may face challenges when their form of identification is inconsistent with their identity. Due to various barriers, only 9% of transgender individuals who wish to update their gender marker on their birth certificate succeed.[12] It is estimated that 260,000 transgender individuals do not possess a government ID correctly reflecting their name and/or gender, representing nearly 20% of the estimated transgender community in the United States.[13] Without updated legal identification, TGNB individuals may have to explain any perceived inconsistency, which can be intrusive and may force the TGNB individual to discuss what may be a private matter to a stranger.

In other cases, an inconsistency in documentation may undermine access to critical services.

By way of example, a transgender woman attends a medical appointment to undergo a fertility workup with a new health care provider. Upon arriving for her appointment, she presents the receptionist with her identification, which indicates a male gender marker, and her health care insurance card. The receptionist reviews both and seeks to confirm the health insurance coverage is active. The receptionist calls the woman back to the counter, explaining the inconsistency between the gender marker on her identification and health care insurance policy may lead the insurer to deny coverage for the medical visit, leaving the full cost of appointment and any tests to be the woman's financial responsibility.

Similar to the foregoing example, a TGNB individual who maintains a medical power of attorney, allowing them to make health care decisions for a spouse or friend, may be prevented from exercising that power if the TGNB individual is asked for identification and the name on the identification and the name listed in the power of attorney are inconsistent. Documents like a medical power of attorney should reference both the TGNB individual's dead or former name and the TGNB individual's chosen name.

A final example comes on the heels of the 2020 presidential election. A transgender woman in North Carolina arrived at her local polling location and provided her legal (male) name to the poll worker. The woman was asked for identification, which reflected her legal name and male gender marker. The request for identification was illegal, as the state's recently enacted voter ID law was not yet in effect. The poll worker persisted, eventually escalating the matter to the chief precinct's judge. While the woman was ultimately allowed to cast her vote, it was intrusive, violative of her right to privacy, and created a potential barrier to exercising her right to vote.

---

[12] James SE, Herman JL, Rankin S, Keisling M, Mottet L, Anafi M. The report of the 2015 U.S. Transgender Survey. Washington, DC: National Center for Transgender Equality, 2016 (https://www.transequality.org/sites/default/files/docs/USTS-Full-Report-FINAL.PDF)

[13] The Potential Impact of Voter Identification Laws on Transgender Voters in the 2020 General Election.

The final example could be replicated in 35 states, which have voter ID laws. As is now the case in North Carolina, an individual attempting to cast their vote who fails to provide identification matching their gender marker on their registration may be turned away.

As individuals encounter medical professionals, health insurance policies, various agencies, or the courtroom, inconsistent identification could create delays or extra costs. To mitigate these challenges, TGNB individuals who are undergoing name changes or birth certificate amendments should retain copies of the documents filed with the relevant court or government office, providing them as needed to help confirm their identity.

Birth Certificates and Gender Markers

TGNB individuals may face challenges obtaining a birth certificate for their child that accurately reflects their own gender identity. For example, even in cases where a delivering parent legally changed their name and identifies as male, some states require that the delivering parent's birth name be listed in the "mother" field on the child's birth certificate. Similarly, while most states have updated their birth certificates to include gender-neutral markers such as "parent" in addition to "mother" and "father," the traditional markers of "mother" and "father" may not be available to TGNB couples; instead, the couple, if perceived as a same-sex couple, will automatically be given markers of "parent" and "parent."

Coincidentally, as this chapter was being written, the *New England Journal of Medicine* published an article in favor of moving gender markers on identification documents "below the line of demarcation." The line of demarcation on documents such as birth certificates separates public information from non-public confidential statistical information. The article's authors argue, among other things, that the gender markers are harmful to a variety of groups (e.g., intersex, non-binary, and transgender) and limit self-identification. From a legal perspective, moving gender markers below the line of demarcation would not only make it simpler for TGNB individuals to more easily assume their true gender identity, but, as the authors argue, the deemphasizing of gender-based distinctions is also in line with the last decade of legal precedent (e.g., same-sex couples' right to marry[14]).

The American Civil Liberties Union (the "ACLU") also listed the removal of gender markers on federal documents as one of their top priorities for President Biden and Vice President Harris to pursue.[15] The ACLU's goal is for the

---

[14] *Obergefell v. Hodges*, 135 S. Ct. 2584 (2015).

[15] https://www.aclu.org/news/lgbt-rights/they-the-people-the-biden-administration-must-go-beyond-repealing-trumps-attacks-on-trans-rights/?initms_aff=nat&initms_chan=soc.&utm_medium=soc.&initms=201220_igstory_ig&utm_source=ig&utm_campaign=&utm_content=201220_lgbtq_igstory&ms_aff=nat&ms_chan=soc.&ms=201220_igstory_ig

11 Legal Considerations

Biden-Harris administration to issue an executive order removing the documentation requirement (e.g., letter from a physician indicating treatment for gender affirmation) that a TGNB individual must provide in order to secure the gender marker that is representative of their identity. The ACLU is also advocating for the addition of the "X" marker option.[16]

The ACA and Health Care Insurance

The ACA, as originally enacted, was revolutionary. For the first time in the history of the United States, all Americans were required to maintain health care insurance and those with preexisting conditions were protected. A lesser publicized provision of the ACA, which is also our focus, provided for the expansion of Medicaid.

Expanding Access

Originally enacted in 1965, Medicaid provided funding to states to assist pregnant women, children, needy families, the disabled, and the elderly. Generally, unemployed applicants whose income was less than 37% of the federal poverty line and employed applicants whose income was less than 63% of the federal poverty line were eligible to receive Medicaid funds.[17]

By contrast, the Medicaid expansion under the ACA required states to expand coverage *to all individuals*, including single head (i.e., childless) households, with incomes below 138% of the federal poverty line.

To put this in perspective, the federal poverty line in 2010 for a one-person household was $10,830, with $3740 added for each additional person within that household. Under the original Medicaid scheme, a single employed parent household with one child would only qualify for benefits if the parent's income was less than $9179.10. Under the ACA, the same family would qualify for Medicaid benefits if they made less than $20,106.60.

How, you ask, was the expansion relevant to TGNB individuals?

In 2014, the Behavioral Risk Factor Surveillance System performed by the Center for Disease Control found that individuals identifying as transgender did much worse in aspects relating to their economic well-being, such as educational attainment, employment, and *poverty status*.[18] Consistent with these findings, a study by the Center for American Progress in 2017 found that lack of insurance within the

---

[16] An "X" marker indicates a sex/gender other than male or female.

[17] https://www.payingforseniorcare.com/federal-poverty-level#2020-Poverty-Guidelines%2D%2D-Annual.

[18] https://www.cdc.gov/brfss/about/index.htm

LGBTQ+ community was highest among transgender individuals.[19] For TGNB individuals without children and without existing health care insurance, the ACA could have provided them with access to medical care. Medical care in this instance could have included something as routine as getting a flu shot to, as it relates to the topic of this book, testing for sexual functioning and, potentially, fertility preservation.

The day President Obama signed the ACA into law, a number of states, several individuals, and the National Federation of Independent Business filed a complaint in federal court alleging that, among other things, the Medicaid expansion was unconstitutional. The case wound its way through the court system, ending at the United State Supreme Court. In *National Federation of Independent Business v. Sebelius*,[20] the Supreme Court ruled that the Medicaid expansion exceeded Congress' constitutional limits. In doing so, the Court struck that portion of the ACA. As a result, Medicaid reverted to its original form, excluding the single head (i.e., childless) households with incomes below 138% of the federal poverty line. The Court's decision left it to Congress to amend the ACA to bring it in line with constitutional limits or for the states themselves to expand Medicaid. Understanding the value of expanding Medicaid to its citizens, 31 states and the District of Columbia expanded their Medicaid programs to cover all individuals with incomes up to 138% of the federal poverty line as of 2016.[21] The Medicaid expansion in these states would disproportionally benefit many TGNB individuals, who experience significantly higher rates of poverty than people who identify as cisgender.[22]

Prohibition of Discrimination and Health Care Insurance Management

As the example in the prior section indicated, gender markers associated with an individual's health care insurance policy that are inconsistent with the individual's identification may curtail access to medical services or potentially lead to the denial of insurance coverage.

In an attempt to address these types of scenarios, the ACA included a provision, Section 1557, prohibiting discrimination based on race, color, national origin, sex, age, and disability in health programs and activities receiving federal financial

---

[19] https://www.americanprogress.org/issues/lgbtq-rights/news/2017/03/22/428970/repealing-affordable-care-act-bad-medicine-lgbt-communities/

[20] *Nat'l Fed'n of Indep. Bus. v. Sebelius*, 567 U.S. 519 (2012).

[21] https://www.americanprogress.org/issues/lgbtq-rights/reports/2016/08/09/142424/the-medicaid-program-and-lgbt-communities-overview-and-policy-recommendations

[22] Transgender people have especially high rates of poverty that create eligibility for Medicaid. Approximately 29.4% of the transgender community experience a state of poverty compared to 13.4% of cis-straight men and 17.8% of cis-straight women. https://williamsinstitute.law.ucla.edu/publications/lgbt-poverty-us/

11 Legal Considerations

assistance.[23, 24] In 2016, the Office for Civil Rights (the "OCR") of the United States Department of Health and Human Services issued a rule clarifying that sex discrimination under Section 1557 included gender identity, which it defined as "one's internal sense of gender, which may be male, female, neither, or a combination of male and female."[25]

In June 2020, the OCR amended its earlier rule, eliminating gender identity as a type of sex discrimination.[26] Notwithstanding the OCR's 2016 or 2020 rules, litigation concerning discrimination against transgender individuals has consistently found that sex discrimination under Section 1557 includes discrimination based on gender identity.[27]

To cement this understanding, the Equality Act, which was passed by the House of Representatives, seeks to amend existing civil rights law—including the Civil Rights Act of 1964, the Fair Housing Act, the Equal Credit Opportunity Act, the Jury Selection and Services Act, and several laws regarding employment with the federal government—to explicitly include sexual orientation and gender identity as protected characteristics.[28]

How many TGNB individuals manage their health care insurance as it relates to fertility preservation and family creation will, once again, come down to prudent planning. This may include delaying changes to identification or gender markers.

For example, a transgender man may opt to delay changing their gender marker on their health insurance coverage and identification until after giving birth. By doing so, insurance claims relating to prenatal care and delivery are less likely to be scrutinized if the patient is identified as female in both the health insurance policy and the identification (i.e., a male patient who delivers a child may be questioned by the insurer or be required to appeal a denial of coverage based solely on the gender marker).[29]

Notwithstanding the interpretation of Section 1557 by federal courts and until the Equality Act is enacted, individuals with inconsistent markers may find it prudent and best practice to request preauthorization for medical treatment. The National Center for Transgender Equality provides guides, form letters, and other resources that may be helpful when requesting preauthorization for medical treatment, such as a cesarean section for a transmasculine person which may not be deemed as medically necessary but psychologically necessary due to genital dysphoria.[30]

---

[23] https://www.congress.gov/bill/111th-congress/house-bill/3590

[24] This prohibition on discrimination was based on the Civil Rights Act of 1964.

[25] https://www.hhs.gov/about/news/2020/06/12/hhs-finalizes-rule-section-1557-protecting-civil-rights-healthcare.html

[26] https://www.federalregister.gov/documents/2020/06/19/2020-11758/nondiscrimination-in-health-and-health-education-programs-or-activities-delegation-of-authority

[27] See *Boyden v. Conlin*, 341 F. Supp. 3d 979 (W.D. Wis. 2018) and *Rumble v. Fairview Health Services*; D.Minn. (2015 WL 1197415).

[28] https://www.congress.gov/bill/116th-congress/house-bill/5/text

[29] This is a perfect example of the discrimination that Section 1557 is meant to address, however, it is a cost-benefit analysis (i.e., have documentation reflect one's true gender identity and potentially receive insurance requests to explain the perceived inconsistency).

[30] https://transequality.org/health-coverage-guide

Conclusion

Fertility preservation and family creation both present unique legal considerations for TGNB individuals. A history of legislative inaction makes it more difficult for individuals from marginalized communities to participate as equals in these practices—even so, such legal challenges can be surmounted or ameliorated with thoughtful planning. In this chapter, we examined how key legislation, legal identification, and access to care create hurdles—and opportunities—for TGNB communities in these domains. We discussed how laws, or the lack thereof, affect access to fertility preservation and parentage for TGNB individuals, and considered how identification on state IDs and birth certificates could lead to legal and social obstacles. Finally, we looked to a point of optimism: the impacts of the Affordable Care Act and the benefits of health care reform for TGNB communities.

Until the legal and social inequities in the fertility preservation and family creation processes are addressed, TGNB communities must often consider the various legal obstacles explored in this chapter. While individuals should seek out legal advice as needed, this chapter provides the legal resources and standards to consider as TGNB individuals embark on their journey. Fertility preservation and family creation are, for many, central pillars of the human experience—no individual should be discouraged from these pursuits on account of their identity.

Chapter 12
Ethical Considerations for Transgender and Non-Binary Reproduction

Lisa Campo-Engelstein and Rebecca M. Permar

Assisted reproductive technologies (ART) have opened the door for many people to pursue genetic parenthood when it was previously not possible for them to do so, including cisgender heterosexual couples with infertility, single individuals, and those in the LGBTQ community [1]. In this chapter, we focus specifically on transgender and non-binary (TGNB) reproduction, providing provide an overview of some of the ethical considerations at play. First, we describe how standard definitions of infertility exclude TGNB individuals, making it more difficult and expensive for them to access ART. Such narrow definitions of infertility uphold cisnormative beliefs about who is deserving of parenthood. Second, we discuss how the highly gendered binary framework upon which reproductive medicine is based marginalizes and erases TGNB individuals. We enumerate some actions fertility clients can take to make TGNB individuals feel welcome. Third, we turn to the high cost of ART, which is a barrier for many people and raises justice concerns. TGNB individuals are especially disadvantaged due to their gender identity and other intersecting marginalized identities Fourth, we examine the challenges for TGNB individuals and clinicians in making decisions about gender-affirming and reproductive care in the face of limited data. Finally, we explore some of the specific issues for TGNB youth, including the question of whether youth should be able to make their own decisions about fertility preservation prior to gender-affirming hormones and surgery.

L. Campo-Engelstein (✉) · R. M. Permar
Institute for Bioethics & Health Humanities, University of Texas Medical Branch, Galveston, TX, USA
e-mail: licampoe@utmb.edu; rmpermar@utmb.edu

© The Author(s), under exclusive license to Springer Nature Switzerland AG 2023
M. B. Moravek, G. de Haan (eds.), *Reproduction in Transgender and Nonbinary Individuals*, https://doi.org/10.1007/978-3-031-14933-7_12

163

Definitions of Infertility

Medical definitions, like medical and scientific terms more broadly, are generally seen as objective. However, as is obvious to us from historical examples like hysteria [2] and drapetomania [3], medical definitions are socially mediated and can embody cultural mores. Contemporary medical definitions are not immune to social influence. In this section, we discuss how the definition of infertility reflects heteronormative, cisgender family structures. A pretty standard definition of infertility is offered by the Centers for Disease Control (CDC): "not being able to get pregnant (conceive) after one year (or longer) of unprotected sex" [4]. Similarly, the World Health Organization (WHO) defines infertility as "the failure to achieve a clinical pregnancy after 12 months or more of regular unprotected sexual intercourse" [5].

There are multiple problematic assumptions in these definitions. First, this definition presumes a couple—and specifically a heterosexual, cisgender couple as we will discuss momentarily—not an individual. Engaging in sexual activity implies that at least two people are involved. Consequently, single people who are not engaging in sexual activity due to lack of a partner cannot be classified as infertile according to this definition precisely because they are single. Furthermore, this definition presumes a long-term, monogamous partner, in order to meet the minimum time frame of 1 year (and some definitions of infertility require more time) of "regular" (a.k.a. regularly scheduled) sexual intercourse. This focus on couples is problematic because we have ways to diagnose individuals as physiologically infertile that do not depend upon a partner (e.g., checking sperm count). The growing field of fertility preservation highlights that individuals recognize the potential for their own physiologic infertility outside of a partnership. For instance, the dramatic growth in egg freezing is mainly driven by cisgender women without partners who are worried about age-related infertility [6].

Second, and most relevant to this chapter, is that standard definitions of infertility do not specify what type of sexual activity they are discussing. Although there are a variety of activities that fall under the umbrella of "sex" and even "intercourse," definitions of fertility do not explicitly state that they are referring to vaginal–penile intercourse since this is the heteronormative standard. Standard definitions of infertility exclude couples who do not engage in vaginal–penile intercourse, which mainly affects individuals in the LGBTQ community. If LGBTQ couples are not engaging in the "right" type of sex, then they cannot be diagnosed as infertile according to standard definitions [7]. There have been cases of cisgender lesbian couples having to "prove" their infertility by paying for intrauterine insemination out-of-pocket for a year to mimic the 1 year of vaginal–penile intercourse standard [8].

In response to these two problematic assumptions, some have argued to expand the definition of infertility beyond physiological infertility to social infertility (also sometimes referred to as relational infertility [9] or structural infertility [10]). Whereas traditional definitions of infertility focus on physiological factors, social infertility acknowledges that one can be fertile or infertile based on one's relationship status [11]. For example, a single person regardless of their sexual orientation and gender identity will always be socially infertile because, on their own and without gamete donation, they lack the two sets of gametes necessary for fertilization. Cisgender, same-sex couples are also socially infertile because they do not, as a couple, have both eggs and sperm. TGNB individuals may also experience social infertility depending upon their partner and also their own fertility status. Some TGNB individuals, for example, may be infertile due to gender affirming surgeries. However, fertility preservation for TGNB individuals is becoming more common and some have banked gametes prior to gender affirming surgeries.

It is important to note that social infertility is not limited to LGBTQ individuals, but also can involve cisgender, heterosexual individuals such as a cis woman who has previous sexual trauma that makes vaginal–penile intercourse painful and a cis man who is sterile from cancer treatment. While the goal of social infertility is to recognize types of infertility that do not adhere to standard definitions, some find this concept problematic because it may lead to a hierarchy of types of infertility, with physiological infertility being elevated over social infertility. Part of the reason for this is that social infertility is typically associated with LGBTQ individuals. Underlying this is the belief that physiological infertility is beyond one's control, whereas people can "choose" whether or not to be socially infertile—an especially troubling claim when directed at LGBTQ individuals. Another concern with social infertility is that it medicalizes sexual orientation and gender identity in order for LGBTQ individuals to receive access to fertility treatment.

Whether or not we choose to distinguish between different types of infertility—social versus physiological—what is important is that definitions of infertility be more inclusive of individuals other than cisgender, heterosexual, monogamous, and long-term couples. While some may disregard this discussion of definitions as mere semantics, much more is at stake here. Medical definitions are powerful: they can shape who "counts" as a patient, who has access to care, and whose treatment is covered by insurance. By reifying social beliefs about normative reproduction, definitions of infertility determine which groups of people are deserving of parenthood. The ethics of TGNB individuals reproducing, particularly their parental "fitness" [12], has been called into question based solely on their gender identity despite lack of evidence that TGNB individuals make "worse" parents than cisgender individuals [13]. Definitions of infertility that only include cisgender individuals reinforce beliefs that TGNB individuals should not reproduce.

Marginalization in the Practice of Fertility Medicine

The embedded cis- and heteronormativity in standard definitions of infertility reflects the orientation of reproductive medicine—as well as cultural conceptions of reproduction more broadly—that is based on a binary in which cisgender women's bodies are the primary focus both because their bodies are assumed to be the location for gestation and because of cultural norms that deeply connect femininity and motherhood [14]. This binary not only minimizes the role cisgender men play in reproduction [15–17], but it also effectively erases TGNB reproduction [18]. This erasure occurs not only on the social level, but also legally and within the bodies of TGNB individuals. For example, in some countries sterilization was, and still is, necessary for changing one's legal gender [19], including countries typically seen as more progressive like Sweden and Finland [12].

The focus on cisgender women's bodies leads fertility clinics to be highly gendered spaces that tend to reinforce dominant gender norms—binary conceptions of femininity and masculinity—and traditional understandings of family formations centered on a cisgender, heterosexual (white, Christian, higher socioeconomic status, and able bodied) couple [20]. For TGNB individuals, entering such a space where they fall outside of the norm can be unsettling [21]. Feelings of discomfort and uncertainty can be magnified when providers are not culturally competent with transgender healthcare, which is common [22]. For example, some providers may not be aware that using gender-specific terminology, like "egg" and "vagina," can be distressing for some TGNB individuals and increase their dysphoria [23]. Even seemingly innocuous things, such as pink forms for egg freezing [24], may cause TGNB individuals to feel out of place and excluded.

Furthermore, clinicians may not know how to talk about TGNB parenthood, especially when they perceive discordance between reproductive role and gender identity (e.g., an individual who contributes sperm and identifies as a mother or a pregnant transmasculine person) [18]. Some TGNB individuals state that clinicians in fertility clinics tended to conflate body parts with gender identity, thereby erasing their TGNB identities and misgendering them and their parental role [21]. Despite the American Society for Reproductive Medicine (ASRM) ethics committee statement that requests for fertility services should be respected regardless of gender identity [25], some TGNB individuals report mistreatment and discrimination by fertility clinics [26]. Such experiences can lead people to seek assistance through informal networks (such as at-home insemination using known donors) rather than continue to pursue treatment within the medical establishment [27].

There are numerous things fertility clients can do to make TGNB individuals feel welcome, from having promotional materials that include various family formations to becoming more educated about transgender healthcare. Additionally, fertility clinics can make their spaces less gendered visually (gender-neutral bathrooms), through language (asking patients for their pronouns), and by stepping outside of the gender binary to acknowledge the range of gender identities (a section of the clinic website dedicated to TGNB reproduction) [26]. A less gendered space would not only benefit TGNB individuals, but all individuals by acknowledging diversity rather than pigeonholing people based on their reproductive organs [28].

Cost of Fertility Treatment

The cost of fertility treatments can be a barrier for all patients, but in this section, we describe some ways in which TGNB individuals are especially disadvantaged due to their gender identity and other intersecting marginalized identities.

Fertility treatments are expensive and can rapidly accumulate. On average, one cycle of IVF costs $12,000, but some estimate a minimum of $66,000 based on the assumption that multiple cycles of IVF will be necessary for a live birth [10]. Most Organisation for Economic Co-operation and Development countries provide universal access and underwriting for ART [29]. In contrast, the United States has a patchwork of coverage through private insurance and state mandates: a little over a quarter of private insurance companies cover ART [30] and 15 states have mandates requiring insurance companies to cover (at least some) ART [31].

Even when people have insurance coverage for ART, there can be caveats limiting access to cisgender, heterosexual married couples who use their gametes (no donor gametes) and gestate the pregnancy (no gestational surrogacy) [32]. These types of restrictions make it more challenging, if not impossible, for TGNB individuals to receive coverage for ART. Moreover, as discussed earlier, TGNB individuals may not meet the cisnormative definition of infertility that a particular insurance company or state is using, which would also exclude them from coverage.

Fertility preservation prior to medical care has not historically been covered by insurance companies because it does not fit within the standard definitions of infertility [33]. In the oncofertility context, some have argued that fertility preservation should be covered for those with anticipated infertility due to medical treatment, such as cancer patients about to undergo potentially sterilizing treatment, since other iatrogenic conditions are generally covered by insurance [34]. The same argument can apply to TGNB individuals: fertility preservation should be covered because gender-affirming care can lead to infertility or sterility. While a handful of states have now expanded their definitions of infertility to include fertility preservation, it is unclear if such coverage extends to TGNB individuals [35]. TGNB individuals have identified the cost of fertility preservation as a major structural barrier to care [36].

While insurance coverage for fertility preservation and other ART for TGNB individuals would increase access, is not a panacea due to systemic disadvantages for and discrimination against marginalized groups. For instance, even in states with infertility mandates, significant racial and socioeconomic disparities can be found among infertility patients [37]. Given that TGNB individuals are more likely to be people of color and living below the poverty line [38], many of them face racial and economic barriers to reproductive care in addition to barriers they may experience because of their gender identity. Additionally, they are more likely to be living in rural areas [38], which can make it more difficult for them to access care, especially if nearby clinics are not trans-inclusive.

That TGNB individuals, as well as others with marginalized identities, face extra hurdles in accessing and affording ART raises justice concerns. Gender identity should not be a consideration in decisions about who receives ART and how much they pay for it. The ASRM [25] and the American Congress of Obstetricians and Gynecologists (ACOG) [39], the two predominant medical organizations in the United States focusing on reproductive healthcare, both assert that it is unethical to discriminate against individuals based on gender identity. Additionally, recent research shows that most people support clinicians helping TGNB individuals have genetic children via ART [40], indicating that the public also endorses equal reproductive rights for TGNB individuals.

Decision-Making despite Uncertainty

The field of TGNB reproduction is quite young, which means there are limited studies to support best practices. This can make clinical decision-making more difficult for TGNB individuals and clinicians. For instance, one review of Medline articles published on the topic of TGNB health through June 2016 found that just 0.9% of all articles focused on TGNB reproduction (only 22 articles), with many of them in the bioethics literature and few clinical studies [41]. While the number of articles on TGNB reproduction seems to have proliferated in the last handful of years, there is still limited specific clinical guidance for TGNB individuals and clinicians from medical organizations like the ASRM, the European Society of Human Reproduction and Embryology, and the World Professional Association for Transgender Health.

However, there does seem to be consensus on two broad recommendations [25, 42, 43] First, clinicians should offer fertility preservation to TGNB individuals prior to gender-affirming medical interventions because gender-affirming surgeries (oophorectomy and orchiectomy) cause sterility and there are limited data on the effects of gender-affirming hormone therapy on reproductive function [44, 45]. Second, clinicians should inform TGNB individuals of the risks of ART (in general and that may be unique to the TGNB population) and the lack of data about long-term outcomes for TGNB individuals and their children.

Informed consent is a cornerstone of clinical practice and medical ethics. In order to give informed consent, individuals must know the risks and benefits of their treatment options and clinicians are responsible for providing this information. Yet when there are such limited data to guide clinical recommendations, clinicians may be unsure how to counsel their patients. The practice of contemporary medicine is grounded in the model of evidence-based medicine, which can leave clinicians caring for TGNB individuals uncertain about how to apply guidelines that do not have a strong scientific grounding [46].

Although uncertainty is ubiquitous in medicine [47], navigating this particular uncertainty may be especially distressing for clinicians since it involves caring for a vulnerable population at the intersection of two significant and sensitive areas: gender identity and reproduction. Decisions at this intersection are deeply personal. For example, whether to postpone gender-affirming care in order to first undergo fertility preservation or whether to go off hormones in order to gestate a pregnancy depends upon one's preferences, physical ability, and values. Clinicians cannot make these types of value-laden decisions for their patients; rather, their role is to paint a clear and accurate clinical picture of the options without hype or false promise and with the explicit acknowledgment of the current limits of our knowledge in the field [48].

Clinician honesty and humility about the state of the field of transgender reproduction fosters a patient/clinician relationship based on trust and respect. TGNB individuals too frequently face discrimination in their clinical encounters [49], which can lead to mistrust and avoidance of healthcare services [50]. A strong patient–physician relationship will make it easier for TGNB individuals to ask questions and feel supported in making what may be difficult and emotional decisions about their gender-affirming and reproductive care based on limited data.

Fertility Preservation Decision-Making in TGNB Youth

As per the ASRM guidelines, TGNB individuals should be offered fertility preservation prior to gender-affirming care [25]. For TGNB youth, this means that they (and their parents/guardians) will have to make decisions about fertility preservation before reaching the legal age of majority. The big question here is: who makes the decision about fertility preservation? Ideally, youth, their parents, and clinicians engage in a shared decision-making process whereby they reach a decision that is acceptable to all. Unfortunately, this is not always the case, so the question emerges of who *ultimately* makes the decision about fertility preservation?

Some parents may believe they should be the ones responsible for this decision because youth do not have the maturity to carefully weigh the relevant factors at play. For instance, some research has shown that transgender youth are not willing to delay gender-affirming hormones in order to preserve fertility [51]—a view some parents may find shortsighted and evidence that youth are not able to carefully weigh all of the factors, both short-term and long-term. Parents may assume make children devalue or do not understand the value of parenthood because they are at a different life stage, one that is typically not focused on reproduction. In contrast, parents may see themselves as better suited to make decisions about fertility preservation given their lived experience as parents.

Furthermore, parents may feel ethically obligated to choose fertility preservation as a way of ensuring their children have a right to an open future: one in which various options, including genetic parenthood, are available to them so that they can make their own decision as adults [52]. Some claim that fertility preservation in pediatric patients should be framed as a rebuttable presumption rather than merely an option because of the importance of maintaining the possibility of future genetic parenthood [53]. The risk-benefit analysis changes, however, when we look at experimental fertility preservation options for prepubertal children, which weakens the imperative to treat fertility preservation as the default option [54]. Another reason parents may want to be the ones making decisions is protecting their children so as to minimize the likelihood of negative feelings like dissatisfaction or regret [55, 56].

While some youth, especially young children, may not have the decision-making capacity and emotional maturity to make informed decisions about fertility preservation, what may also be a play is a difference in values between youth and their parents. Some research shows that the parents of TGNB individuals' youth rate genetic parenthood much higher than their children and that for many of the TGNB individuals interested in parenthood, they preferred adoption to genetic parenthood [57]. However, without knowledge of high costs and long waits [58] for adoption as well as the fact that some states and adoption agencies discriminate against LGBTQ individuals [59], youth may not realize the challenges they may face with alternative family building options.

Nonetheless, there are strong reasons for deferring to youth, especially adolescents, for these decisions. The overarching one is that respecting patient autonomy is a central tenet of medical ethics. Yet, certain individuals and groups are exempted from this because they are seen as lacking decision-making capacity. In the United States, minors (those under the age of 18) fall into this category and are not generally legally able to give valid consent to medical treatment. The American Academy of Pediatrics (AAP), however, asserts that youth should be involved in the medical decision-making process "to the extent of their capacity" [60]. Influential research in the field of child psychology shows that children as young as age 9 can meaningfully participate in medical decision-making and that adolescents at age 14 are just as competent as adults in key criteria for medical decision-making [61]. Even if one is skeptical that children so young have decision-making capacity, it is no doubt clear that cognitive and emotional development varies among youth, leaving open the possibility that some may have the maturity to make their own medical decisions before reaching the legal age of majority, whereas others may not. In fact, there have been court cases where individuals under 18 were recognized as having the capacity to make their own medical decisions [62]. Furthermore, the AAP Committee of Bioethics guidelines state that minors who are deemed to have decision-making capacity are entitled to the same degree of autonomy as adult patients [60].

Another reason to defer to youth is that those under 18 are legally allowed to confidentially consent to and receive treatment for sensitive issues like reproductive healthcare, sexually transmitted infections, mental health, and substance use in most states [63]. It seems inconsistent to allow youth to make their own medical decisions about other aspects of their reproductive health (with the notable exception of abortion in some states) but to treat fertility preservation differently. Reproductive decision-making is typically seen as a deeply personal and private matter that is best left up to individuals themselves rather than others. Parental decision-making about fertility preservation does not always mirror the youth's wishes [64]. As treatment decisions shift from clear-cut (performing lifesaving surgery) to more subjective (undergoing fertility preservation), youth's voices should play a more significant role so that these decisions reflect their values [65]. Turning to the preferences of trans youth, one study found that 72% of TGNB teenagers wanted to make a decision about fertility preservation themselves, without parental involvement [51].

An important component of respecting patient autonomy is the right to bodily integrity. In medicine, patients' negative right—the right to noninterference—is almost universal; exceptions are generally limited to the spread of serious infectious diseases. This negative right is so foundational that performing a procedure on someone against their wishes is considered an assault [66]. Situations where the parents are advocating for fertility preservation while the youth is reluctant to run the risk of the youth being pressured or coerced. One study found that almost 25% of TGNB youth felt pressured by their family to have genetic children and 28% said not having genetic children would be a disappointment for the family [67]. Given our pronatalist culture, it is important for children to recognize that there are alternative family formation to genetic parenthood and that non-parenthood is also an acceptable choice [68].

Clearly, there are times when parents are justifiably paternalistic and mandate their child undergo a medical procedure against the child's wishes; childhood vaccinations are one example. Yet what differentiates vaccinations from fertility preservation is that they are a standard part of childhood care that are potentially lifesaving and have extremely high success rates whereas fertility preservation is elective (at least in the sense that it is not lifesaving) and there is no guarantee that it will result in genetic children. In addition to concerns about violating bodily integrity, performing unwanted fertility preservation goes against the principle of nonmaleficence. Some fertility preservation procedures are quite invasive (e.g., transvaginal ultrasounds), which people of all ages may find distressing, but it may be worse for younger people, especially if they are not sexually active. Furthermore, fertility preservation procedures like transvaginal ultrasounds and hormonal stimulation can exacerbate gender dysphoria for TGNB youth, which can adversely affect their mental health [69].

Whereas negative rights in medicine are almost absolute, positive rights—the right to something—are limited. In situations where the youth wants fertility preservation, but the parents are objecting, it is unlikely that the youth would be able to undergo fertility preservation. First, in many states, minors need parental consent for fertility preservation and even where this law does not apply, clinics may be hesitant to provide such a service to minors without parental involvement [70]. Second, as previously discussed, ART is expensive, and most minors would not be able to afford fertility preservation on their own.

If there is a disagreement between youth and their parents about whether to pursue fertility preservation, clinicians may be able to mediate to uncover the source of the disagreement. Youth may be scared or may not fully understand the procedure, so clinicians should not accept a hasty refusal [71]. Some research shows low utilization of fertility preservation by TGNB youth [72]. To address these concerns, youth should ideally have multiple conversations with their parents and their multidisciplinary healthcare team [73]. Given the heightened vulnerability of TGNB youth—they are at greater risk than cisgender youth for substance use, physical and sexual violence, mental health issues, transactional sex, and involvement with the criminal justice system [74, 75]—it is imperative that they have a trusting and supportive relationship with their healthcare team, particularly if they do not have strong family support.

Conclusion

In this chapter, we have discussed various ethical considerations at play in transgender reproduction. A couple of common themes have emerged. First is the importance of inclusivity. TGNB individuals are excluded from standard definitions of infertility, erased from highly gendered fertility clinics, and denied the same level of access to ART. As a matter of social justice, we need to ensure that TGNB individuals have the same rights to ART and are equally welcomed as all other groups. Second is the significance of the patient/clinician relationship. The field of transgender reproduction, as well as the field of transgender health more broadly, is relatively young and therefore data upon which to base clinical standards are limited. Having a trustworthy and supportive relationship with clinicians is essential for TGNB individuals to make informed decisions about their care in the face of limited evidence. Similarly, a trustworthy and supportive relationship is crucial for TGNB youth who are especially vulnerable and may not be cognitively and emotionally prepared to make difficult decisions. As the field of transgender reproduction continues to grow and evolve some ethical concerns may be mitigated while new ethical considerations may emerge. We should continue to examine the ethical issues in this field so that TGNB individuals can receive quality healthcare that focuses on inclusivity and compassion.

References

1. Gürtin ZB, Faircloth C. Conceiving contemporary parenthood: imagining, achieving and accounting for parenthood in new family forms. Anthropol Med. 2018;25(3):243–8.
2. Tasca C, Rapetti M, Carta MG, Fadda B. Women and hysteria in the history of mental health. Clin Pract Epidemiol Ment Health. 2012;8:110–9.
3. Naragon MD. Communities in motion: Drapetomania, work and the development of African-American slave cultures. Slavery Abolition. 1994;15(3):63–87.
4. Centers for Disease Control and Prevention. Infertility FAQs 2019. https://www.cdc.gov/reproductivehealth/infertility/index.htm.
5. Zegers-Hochschild F, Adamson GD, de Mouzon J, Ishihara O, Mansour R, Nygren K, et al. International Committee for Monitoring Assisted Reproductive Technology (ICMART) and the World Health Organization (WHO) revised glossary of ART terminology, 2009. Fertil Steril. 2009;92(5):1520–4.

6. Inhorn MC, Birenbaum-Carmeli D, Birger J, Westphal LM, Doyle J, Gleicher N, et al. Elective egg freezing and its underlying socio-demography: a binational analysis with global implications. Reprod Biol Endocrinol. 2018;16(1):70.
7. Mamo L. Queering reproduction: achieving pregnancy in the age of technoscience, vol. xi. Durham, NC: Duke University Press; 2007.
8. Mazzola J. Lesbian couples sue N.J., say fertility laws discriminate against them. NJcom. 2016 August 8.
9. Murphy J. Should lesbians count as infertile couples? Antilesbian discrimination in assisted reproduction. In: Purdy ADLM, editor. Embodying bioethics: recent feminist advances. Landam, Md: Rowman & Littlefield; 1999.
10. Centanni C. Using ART to make a baby: how Rhode Island's insurance coverage mandate is preventing same-sex couples from having biological children. Roger Williams University Law Review. 2019;24(2):331–58.
11. Lo W, Campo-Engelstein L. Expanding the clinical definition of infertility to include socially infertile individuals and couples. In: Campo-Engelstein L, Burcher P, editors. Reproductive ethics II. Springer International Publishing AG; 2018. p. 71–83.
12. Honkasalo J. Unfit for parenthood? Compulsory sterilization and transgender reproductive justice in Finland. J Int Women's Stud. 2018;20(1):40–52.
13. Murphy TF. The ethics of helping transgender men and women have children. Perspect Biol Med. 2010;53(1):46–60.
14. Marsh M, Ronner W. The empty cradle: infertility in America from colonial times to the present. Baltimore: Johns Hopkins University Press; 1996.
15. Daniels C. Exposing men: the science and politics of male reproduction. New York: Oxford University Press; 2006.
16. Barnes LW. Conceiving masculinity: male infertility, medicine, and identity. Philadelphia, PA: Temple University Press; 2014.
17. Almeling R. GUYnecology: the missing science of men's reproductive health. Berkeley: University of California Press; 2020.
18. Hoffkling A, Obedin-Maliver J, Sevelius J. From erasure to opportunity: a qualitative study of the experiences of transgender men around pregnancy and recommendations for providers. BMC Pregnancy Childbirth. 2017;17(2).
19. Ho V, Sherqueshaa S, Zheng D. The forced sterilization of transgender and gender non-conforming people in Singapore. LGBTQ POLICY. 2016;6:53.
20. Bell AV. Misconception: social class and infertility in America. Rutgers University Press; 2014.
21. Epstein R. Space invaders: queer and trans bodies in fertility clinics. Sexualities. 2018;21(7):1039–58.
22. Sumerau JE, Mathers LAB. America through transgender eyes. Lanham, MD: Rowman & Littlefield Publishers; 2019.
23. Armuand G, Dhejne C, Olofsson JI, Rodriguez-Wallberg KA. Transgender men's experiences of fertility preservation: a qualitative study. Hum Reprod. 2017;32(2):383–90.
24. Payne JG, Erbenius T. Conceptions of transgender parenthood in fertility care and family planning in Sweden: from reproductive rights to concrete practices. Anthropol Med. 2018;25(3):329–43.
25. Access to fertility services by transgender persons: an ethics committee opinion. Fertil Steril. 2015;104(5):1111–5.
26. James-Abra S, Tarasoff LA, Green D, Epstein R, Anderson S, Marvel S, et al. Trans people's experiences with assisted reproduction services: a qualitative study. Hum Reprod. 2015;30(6):1365–74.
27. Charter R, Ussher JM, Perz J, Robinson K. The transgender parent: experiences and constructions of pregnancy and parenthood for transgender men in Australia. Int J Transgend. 2018;19(1):64–77.
28. Moseson H, Zazanis N, Goldberg E, Fix L, Durden M, Stoeffler A, et al. The imperative for transgender and gender nonbinary inclusion: beyond women's health. Obstet Gynecol. 2020;135(5):1059–68.

29. Adashi EY, Dean LA. Access to and use of infertility services in the United States: framing the challenges. Fertil Steril. 2016;105(5):1113–8.
30. Management SfHR. 2014 employee benefits: an overview of employee benefit offerings in the US. VA: Author Alexandria; 2014.
31. Dupree JM, Dickey RM, Lipshultz LI. Inequity between male and female coverage in state infertility laws. Fertil Steril. 2016.
32. Liu JJ, Adashi E, editors. Selective justice : state mandates for assisted reproductive technology and reproductive justice 2013.
33. Basco D, Campo-Engelstein L, Rodriguez S. Insuring against infertility: expanding state infertility mandates to include fertility preservation technology for cancer patients. J Law Med Ethics. 2010;38(4):832–9.
34. Campo-Engelstein L. Consistency in insurance coverage for iatrogenic conditions resulting from cancer treatment including fertility preservation. J Clin Oncol. 2010;28(8):1284–6.
35. Kyweluk MA, Reinecke J, Chen D. Fertility preservation legislation in the United States: potential implications for transgender individuals. LGBT Health. 2019;6(7):331–4.
36. Tishelman AC, Sutter ME, Chen D, Sampson A, Nahata L, Kolbuck VD, et al. Health care provider perceptions of fertility preservation barriers and challenges with transgender patients and families: qualitative responses to an international survey. J Assist Reprod Genet. 2019;36(3):579–88.
37. Galic I, Negris O, Warren C, Brown D, Bozen A, Jain T. Disparities in access to fertility care: who's in and who's out. F&S Rep. 2020;
38. Crissman HP, Berger MB, Graham LF, Dalton VK. Transgender demographics: a household probability sample of US adults, 2014. Am J Public Health. 2017;107(2):213–5.
39. Committee opinion no. 512: health care for transgender individuals. Obstet Gynecol. 2011;118(6):1454–8.
40. Goldman RH, Kaser DJ, Missmer SA, Farland LV, Scout ARK, et al. Fertility treatment for the transgender community: a public opinion study. J Assist Reprod Genet. 2017;34(11):1457–67.
41. Review of the transgender literature: where do we go from here? Transgend Health. 2017;2(1):119–28.
42. European society of human reproduction and embryology. Female Fertility Preservation. 2020.
43. World Professional Association for Transgender Health. Standards of care for the health of transsexual, transgender, and gender nonconforming people. 7th ed 2011.
44. Moravek MB, Kinnear HM, George J, Batchelor J, Shikanov A, Padmanabhan V, et al. Impact of exogenous testosterone on reproduction in transgender men. Endocrinology. 2020;161:3.
45. Jiang DD, Swenson E, Mason M, Turner KR, Dugi DD, Hedges JC, et al. Effects of estrogen on spermatogenesis in transgender women. Urology. 2019;132:117–22.
46. Shuster SM. Uncertain expertise and the limitations of clinical guidelines in transgender healthcare. J Health Soc Behav. 2016;57(3):319–32.
47. Politi MC, Han PKJ, Col NF. Communicating the uncertainty of harms and benefits of medical interventions. Med Decis Mak. 2007;27(5):681–95.
48. Patient access to experimental treatments. Nuffield Council on Bioethics; 2018.
49. Rodriguez A, Agardh A, Asamoah BO. Self-reported discrimination in health-care settings based on recognizability as transgender: a cross-sectional study among transgender U.S. citizens. Arch Sex Behav. 2018;47(4):973–85.
50. Lerner JE, Martin JI, Gorsky GS. More than an apple a day: factors associated with avoidance of doctor visits among transgender, gender nonconforming, and nonbinary people in the USA. Sexuality Research and Social Policy. 2020.
51. Persky RW, Gruschow SM, Sinaii N, Carlson C, Ginsberg JP, Dowshen NL. Attitudes toward fertility preservation among transgender youth and their parents. J Adolesc Health. 2020;67(4):583–9.
52. Feinberg J. The child's right to an open future. In: Aiken W, LaFollette H, editors. Whose child? Totowa, NJ: Rowman & Littlefield; 1980. p. 124–53.

12 Ethical Considerations for Transgender and Non-Binary Reproduction

53. McDougall R. The ethics of fertility preservation for paediatric cancer patients: from offer to rebuttable presumption. Bioethics. 2015;29(9):639–45.
54. McDougall RJ, Gillam L, Delany C, Jayasinghe Y. Ethics of fertility preservation for prepubertal children: should clinicians offer procedures where efficacy is largely unproven? J Med Ethics. 2018;44(1):27–31.
55. Jayasuriya S, Peate M, Allingham C, Li N, Gillam L, Zacharin M, et al. Satisfaction, disappointment and regret surrounding fertility preservation decisions in the paediatric and adolescent cancer population. J Assist Reprod Genet. 2019;36(9):1805–22.
56. Harris RM, Kolaitis IN, Frader JE. Ethical issues involving fertility preservation for transgender youth. J Assist Reprod Genet. 2020;37(10):2453–62.
57. Chiniara LN, Viner C, Palmert M, Bonifacio H. Perspectives on fertility preservation and parenthood among transgender youth and their parents. Arch Dis Child. 2019;104(8):739–44.
58. Child Welfare Information Gateway. Planning for adoption: knowing the costs and resources. Washington, DC: U.S. Department of Health and Human Services, Children's Bureau; 2016.
59. Stack L. Texas bill would let adoption agencies reject families on religious grounds. New York Times. 2017; May 11
60. Informed consent, parental permission, and assent in pediatric practice. Committee on Bioethics, American Academy of Pediatrics. Pediatrics. 1995;95(2):314–7.
61. Weithorn LA, Campbell SB. The competency of children and adolescents to make informed treatment decisions. Child Dev. 1982;53(6):1589–98.
62. Blake V. Minors' refusal of life-saving therapies. Virtual Mentor. 2012;14(10):792–6.
63. Weddle M, Kokotailo PK. Confidentiality and consent in adolescent substance abuse: an update. Virtual Mentor. 2005;7:3.
64. Johnson EK, Finlayson C. Preservation of fertility potential for gender and sex diverse individuals. Transgend Health. 2016;1(1):41–4.
65. McCabe MA. Involving children and adolescents in medical decision making: developmental and clinical considerations. J Pediatr Psychol. 1996;21(4):505–16.
66. Schoendorff v. Society of New York Hosp., 105 N.E. 92, 93 (N.Y. 1914).
67. Strang JF, Jarin J, Call D, Clark B, Wallace GL, Anthony LG, et al. Transgender youth fertility attitudes questionnaire: measure development in nonautistic and autistic transgender youth and their parents. J Adolesc Health. 2018;62(2):128–35.
68. Riggs DW. An examination of 'just in case' arguments as they are applied to fertility preservation for transgender people. The Reproductive Industry: Intimate Experiences and Global Processes. 2019:69.
69. Kyweluk MA, Sajwani A, Chen D. Freezing for the future: transgender youth respond to medical fertility preservation. Int J Transgend. 2018;19(4):401–16.
70. Fertility preservation and reproduction in cancer patients. Fertil Steril. 2005;83(6):1622–8.
71. Shnorhavorian M, Johnson R, Shear SB, Wilfond BS. Responding to adolescents with cancer who refuse sperm banking: when "no" should not be the last word. J Adolesc Young Adult Oncol. 2011;1(3):114–7.
72. Nahata L, Tishelman AC, Caltabellotta NM, Quinn GP. Low fertility preservation utilization among transgender youth. J Adolesc Health. 61(1):40–4.
73. Chen D, Simons L. Ethical considerations in fertility preservation for transgender youth: a case illustration. Clin Pract Pediatr Psychol. 2018;6(1):93.
74. Giordano S. Lives in a chiaroscuro. Should we suspend the puberty of children with gender identity disorder? J Med Ethics. 2008;34(8):580–4.
75. Cochran BN, Stewart AJ, Ginzler JA, Cauce AM. Challenges faced by homeless sexual minorities: comparison of gay, lesbian, bisexual, and transgender homeless adolescents with their heterosexual counterparts. Am J Public Health. 2002;92(5):773–7.

Chapter 13
Creating Inclusive, Gender Affirming Clinical Environments

Jen Hastings, Ben Geilhufe, J. M. Jaffe, Jenna Rapues, and Colt St. Amand

Background

A gender affirming clinical environment is essential to providing healthcare for all genders. While recognizing that language is limiting and imperfect, this book uses the terms transgender, nonbinary, and intersex (TGNBI) to acknowledge the wide breadth of gender experience outside of endosex (Endosex: description of someone whose primary and sexual characteristics are expected for the male or female sex,

---

J. Hastings (✉)
Department of Family and Community Medicine, University of California San Francisco, Santa Cruz, CA, USA
e-mail: jen@coho.org

B. Geilhufe
UCSF Child and Adolescent Gender Center, San Francisco, CA, USA

Santa Clara University, Santa Clara, CA, USA

Private Practice, Santa Cruz, CA, USA

J. M. Jaffe
Lyon-Martin Health Services, San Francisco, CA, USA

Trans Health Consulting, LLC, San Francisco, CA, USA
e-mail: jjaffe@lyon-martin.org

J. Rapues
San Francisco Department of Public Health, Behavioral Health Services, Gender Health SF, San Francisco, CA, USA
e-mail: jenna.rapues@sfdph.org

C. St. Amand
Department of Psychology, University of Houston, Houston, TX, USA

Department of Family Medicine, Mayo Clinic, Rochester, MN, USA
e-mail: st.amand.colton@mayo.edu

© The Author(s), under exclusive license to Springer Nature Switzerland AG 2023
M. B. Moravek, G. de Haan (eds.), *Reproduction in Transgender and Nonbinary Individuals*, https://doi.org/10.1007/978-3-031-14933-7_13

or simply, someone who is not intersex) cis gender people, including gender diverse, gender expansive, gender fluid, genderqueer, agender, metagender, third gender, and xenogender people, and more. Of note, intersex individuals can identify as any gender and may or may not consider themselves transgender or gender diverse.

Transgender patients regularly report significant discrimination in healthcare systems and avoid seeking care because of fear of discrimination [1, 2]. According to the 2015 US Transgender Discrimination Survey, 33% of respondents recalled at least one negative experience in healthcare due to their transgender identity. TGNBI patients of color and with disabilities reported even higher rates of negative experiences. Nearly one-third of respondents shared they had not disclosed their gender to any of their healthcare providers. Some patients reported avoiding medical settings completely due to the fear of gender-related discrimination, or the stress of having to educate their own healthcare staff about their bodies and their medical needs. Common experiences of discrimination identified by TGNBI patients include refusal of services by medical professionals due to their gender identity, being misgendered during medical appointments, and being denied insurance coverage for gender-related medical care [3, 4]. These experiences can reinforce internalized transphobia and increase minority stress [5] and increase the likelihood that TGNBI patients will avoid seeking medical care in the future [1].

Accessing reproductive healthcare may be especially traumatic for TGNBI patients, as reproductive care has historically been ignored as irrelevant, forcibly controlled, or accessible only through "women's healthcare." In the past, many countries, including the United States, required the removal of gonads as part of gender transition [6, 7]. Additionally, involuntary sterilization has been forced on TGNBI individuals, and especially people of color [8]. Genital surgeries to "normalize" genitalia (i.e., create a genital appearance consistent with that expected of an endosex male or female) are still forced upon intersex children, often resulting in loss of fertility and sexual sensation. It was not until 2014 that the World Professional Association of Transgender Health formally recognized the reproductive rights of transgender and intersex persons [9].

Using the term "reproductive health" rather than "women's health" to refer to gynecological and reproductive healthcare supports persons of all genders to access necessary care, such as pap smears, pelvic exams, prenatal, pregnancy, abortion, and menopausal care. In gender care historically there has been the mistaken assumption that a person's gender embodiment goals would align with their gender within a binary framework: that all women want to have a vagina and all men want a phallus, and with no acknowledgment of genders beyond the binary. We now recognize that gender is truly distinct from one's anatomy. For example, a woman may be at ease with her testes, scrotum, and penis, while another woman may want to have affirming procedures to create a vagina; a man may want to retain his vagina and uterus or may want a surgical phalloplasty or metoidioplasty; and it has become surgically possible to have phalloplasty or metoidioplasty and retain the vagina and uterus (likewise have vaginoplasty and retain the penis) whether or not one's gender is nonbinary or gender diverse. Focusing on sexual and reproductive organs present, the current sex hormone balance, and the medical care needed, rather than the assumed gender of those receiving the medical care, create a safer and inclusive environment for TGNBI individuals, and, in fact, for all individuals. Reconceptualizing "women's health" as "reproductive health" for all genders requires intentionality and a keen awareness of the components of gender inclusive and affirming care [10–12].

The process of identifying and implementing changes to create a model gender affirming environment requires clinic-wide engagement from the first patient contact with the scheduler to the last patient contact with the healthcare provider, lab technician, or biller. A collaborative team approach is considered most effective, with engaged representatives from each part of the clinic, forming a dedicated working group [13]. Ideally, this workgroup should include administrators; reception/registration, IT and billing staff; medical assistants; and providers.

Trials of small changes through iterative, continuous quality improvement, such as PDSA (Plan, Do, Study, Act), provide an evidence-based approach that allows for small but important steps in the adoption of these new clinic processes while harnessing staff desires for change and facilitating spread throughout the organization [13]. Areas to focus on for improvement include registration, intake, billing, and electronic medical record documentation. Establishing and empowering a TGNBI Community Advisory Board to work alongside the working group is a valuable organizational best practice. This larger group can be responsible for vetting emerging best practices and changes in language as well as conducting community and clinic needs assessments, patient feedback, and periodic audits to ensure quality [14, 15].

An integrated behavioral health system, a patient navigator program consisting of TGNBI navigators, and medical–legal partnerships are patient-centered improvements that should be considered integral to the experience and quality of a gender care program. Behavioral health providers on site can facilitate timely counseling and provide needed letters for referrals, including accessing gender affirming medical and surgical interventions and related referrals. Navigators can support patients with many aspects of gender care including negotiating the healthcare system, prescriptions, insurance appeals, name and gender change processes, and support with other social and legal needs such as housing and employment. Medical–legal partnerships can provide support for more complex legal issues as well as legal name and gender changes.

Creating a gender affirming clinic culture and inclusive clinical environment involves changes in language, non-discrimination policies, physical spaces, electronic health records, intake processes, telehealth, billing and insurance, marketing, and staff-wide training. We will now review each of these aspects. The creation and maintenance of an inclusive, gender affirming clinical environment is a dynamic process that demands openness and ongoing assessment as this field continues to change rapidly.

Affirming Language

Staff need to be aware of the importance of language as it is foundational to providing appropriate gender care. Initial contact with staff impacts patients' perception of safety. Patients should be greeted with warmth, regardless of perceived gender identity or expression. When staff use affirming language, demonstrate acceptance, discuss confidentiality, and have protocols specifically to create safety, patients are more willing to share accurate information about themselves, their lives, and their health priorities and are more likely to return to the clinic for future care [16–20].

Gender affirming language and correct name/pronoun use are important throughout the visit. TGNBI patients report that their chosen pronouns are often ignored or not used in clinical settings profoundly impacting their experience. When patients are referred to with a wrong name, pronoun, honorific (e.g., Mr.), term of endearment (e.g., sweetheart), term of address (e.g., lady), or otherwise gendered language, this is known as misgendering. Not recognizing a patient's gender identity, chosen/affirmed name, or pronouns can be traumatic to the patient and harmful to a healing and trusted clinical relationship [21, 22]. The frequency of experiences of being misgendered is positively correlated with depression and suicidality [23]. Misgendering is harmful.

An important principle in correct name and pronouns use is to *ask* the patient how they would like to be addressed. A patient's pronouns should not be assumed based on the name on the chart, physical appearance, voice pitch, or previous visits. Name, pronouns, and gender identity can change over time. Some patients may have multiple gender identities and multiple sets of pronouns, including nongendered pronouns such as they/them. Patient encounters should begin with a nongendered greeting, such as "Hello!" or "Welcome!" until the patient's name and pronouns are confirmed. "Is this the name you generally use?" "What pronouns do you use?" and "Do you have an additional name associated with your chart or insurance?" can follow. It is recommended that all staff that interact with the patient share both their name and pronouns. For example, "Hello, my name is Dr. Sang, my pronouns are they, them. How can I assist you today?" or, "Good morning, my name is Rand, and my pronouns are she, her. How can I help you today?" Adding pronouns to one's greeting and using pronouns such as "they/them," may feel awkward initially, for those new to these practices. Over time and with repetition, this becomes a natural part of speech.

Including staff pronouns in all physical or virtual locations that display the staff person's name is a best practice. Examples include name tags, lab coats, clinic badges, email signatures, and other written correspondence. Buttons with personal pronouns are also recommended and appreciated by patients. See (Fig. 13.1) "name tag and pronoun buttons (Fig. 13.2) "Pronouns Matter."

Given that affirming language is evolving so rapidly and can differ by geographical location and age of TGNBI patients, it is important that the workgroup regularly check with TGNBI staff, patients, and community board members regarding current

13 Creating Inclusive, Gender Affirming Clinical Environments

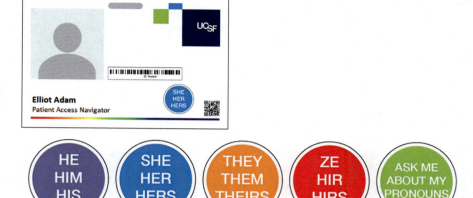

Fig. 13.1 Examples of "Name tag and pronoun buttons" UCSF LGBT Resource Center (with permission)

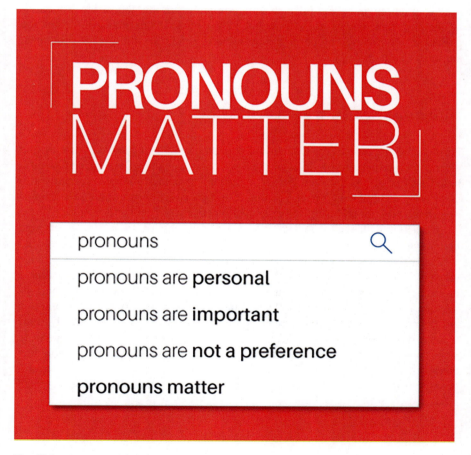

Fig. 13.2 "Pronouns Matter" UCSF LGBT Resource Center (with permission)

and local terminology. The section on collecting information on SOGI (sexual orientation, gender identity, and sometimes referred to as SOGIE, with the addition of gender expression) will discuss the language used for data collection and reporting. Note that the language currently recommended for collecting this federal data is experienced as outdated and triggering for some.

Handling Mistakes

Mistakes are inevitable and should be expected. Staff may use incorrect pronouns, use an old or former name, or make assumptions about gender and anatomy. When a mistake is made, a short, clear apology followed by accurate language use is recommended. For example, "I apologize for using the wrong pronouns/name, [patient's chosen name]. I know your pronouns are [patient's accurate pronouns]. I will do better moving forward." Do not include a personal reflection on how the process feels or how difficult it is (i.e., "This is so difficult for me but I'm trying my hardest!"). Hearing that it is difficult for a provider to use accurate language can inadvertently communicate that the patient's identity is not important and is not paramount in the clinical relationship. Center the patient in the apology by apologizing, honoring their accurate name/pronouns, and then move on.

Hiring and Non-Discrimination Policies

Hiring staff that reflects the diversity of the community being served and ensuring clear non-discrimination policies are the foundation of gender affirming, community-based healthcare. Along with gender inclusion, an organizational commitment to addressing and reducing racial, economic, and social inequities should be adopted as a framework for all hiring and employer practices.

Interacting with gender diverse staff can create a sense of connection, safety, and belonging for TGNBI patients. The clinic's non-discrimination policy should explicitly protect gender identity and expression for both patients and staff; include relevant language specific to local or state non-discrimination laws; and outline a procedure to address transphobia or discrimination, both experienced and witnessed. The policy should also clearly state that there are no gender expression requirements for patients to be protected by this policy [24, 25]. Historically, trans women were required to wear "female clothing" and trans men were required to wear "male clothing" as part of the "Real Life Test," in order to access hormone therapies and surgical procedures [26]. This is now acknowledged as a harmful practice and clinics should make it clear that they do not follow these outdated guidelines.

Staff Training/Staff Considerations

Cultivating a Gender Affirming Clinic Culture

One of the most important aspects of creating a gender inclusive clinical culture is ongoing, staff-wide training. A patient's experience is shaped by each and every staff member with whom they interact. All staff, including staff such as administrators and IT, need to be trained on gender affirming practices and embody a humble disposition when it comes to the gender welcoming culture.

The lack of provider and staff education is a key barrier to providing competent healthcare for transgender and nonbinary patients [27]. Providers and staff avoid gender-related topics for fear of making mistakes and unconscious biases. The assumptions that endosex and cisgender are normal, and that intersex and/or gender diverse persons are, by comparison, abnormal, are unrecognized beliefs that increase stigma and discrimination in healthcare settings for TGNBI patients [4].

When staff are trained on the specific components of gender affirming care, studies show that provider confidence increases significantly and patient distress decreases [28, 29]. Clinicians, academicians, and advocates recommend adding gender care training to graduate education programs, as well as requiring ongoing continuing education in gender care. Research has identified that ongoing training (at least 3 hours or more) offers more sustainable change than single lectures; creates greater access to competent staff; and can help dismantle healthcare disparities affecting TGNBI patients [29, 30]. By training all staff and implementing gender affirmative policies and procedures, a clear message is sent to patients: we serve all genders here.

Critical Components of Ongoing Staff Training

This section presents a brief overview of some of the critical components of ongoing gender affirming staff training. While all staff need training on the importance of gender affirming care and accurate language use, certain employees may require additional role-specific training. For example, HR staff may need additional information about state and federal non-discrimination law, and how to create gender inclusive job announcements and applications; front office staff may need specific training on SOGI data collection; mental health providers will need training on trauma-informed gender affirming care, how to conceptualize and address the high rates of co-occurring mental health conditions and how to advocate for and support patients with their individual goals accessing medical and surgical care; medical providers will need in-depth training on trauma-informed physical exams, how to prescribe hormone therapy, various techniques of gender affirming surgery, how to manage post-op complications, how to counsel patients on what is needed for a healthy, post-operative recovery, how to check in with patients to assess experiences of misgendering when accessing care at their clinic, and how to provide primary and reproductive healthcare given the diversity of TGNBI anatomy and physiology.

At a minimum, the critical components of gender affirming staff training are thought to include Foundations of Gender, the Gender Affirmative Model, Nongendered Language, Provider Bias, Gender inclusive Clinic Space, and Policies and Procedures. The following is a brief overview of each section. For specific resources on developing and disseminating clinic-wide training, see Appendix 2: Training and Other Resources for Providers.

Foundations of Gender

The Foundations of Gender includes language and terminology, differentiation of gender and sexual orientation, cultural sensitivity, and an exploration of gender from both a cross-cultural and historical perspective. Gender Spectrum, an education and advocacy organization, identifies three Dimensions of Gender: (1) Body—physical sex characteristics including chromosomes, relative levels of sex hormones post-puberty, internal genitalia and external genitalia, or components of "sex designated (or assigned) at birth;" (2) Social Gender—gender expression, or how we "do" gender, including culturally based gender roles, clothing, mannerisms; and (3) Gender Identity—our internal core sense of self, a name we use to describe our gender. Examples of gender identities include nonbinary, demi-boy, genderqueer, gender fluid, woman, man metagender, xenogender, and so much more. A person's gender identity may not align with their sex characteristics or sex designated at birth [31].

The Gender Affirmative Clinical Model

Providers working in reproductive health should have knowledge about the interdisciplinary Gender Affirmative Clinical Model and be trained in trauma-informed care [32]. It is sobering to note that the field of transgender health was created by and continues to be dominated by cisgender professionals, and that well-meaning cisgender providers without adequate training have caused harm through lack of understanding and sensitivity needed in the care of TGNBI people. Providers should be versed in the informed consent model for hormone therapy and surgery, hormone therapy, gender affirming surgeries, and how hormones and surgeries may impact reproductive capability [33, 34]. A provider must be knowledgeable and ready to support a vast array of reproductive possibilities. Advances in surgeries have created a wide variety of possible sex anatomies, such as a body with testes and a vulva, a body with one ovary and no uterus, and a body with a penis and uterus. Providers must also develop cultural sensitivity regarding the distress that

13 Creating Inclusive, Gender Affirming Clinical Environments

gender diverse patients may experience from reproductive procedures. For example, the process of obtaining sperm may cause harmful distress for a patient with testes, while experiencing an intravaginal ultrasound prior to egg extraction may cause harmful distress for a patient with a vagina. Staff should collaborate with each patient to identify sources of distress and how to decrease or avoid it, if at all possible. An abdominal or a rectal ultrasound, for example, may be alternative options for the patient who experiences distress with an intravaginal ultrasound. Gender care often requires providers to advocate on behalf of their patients. Providers should be familiar with health insurance, legal matters, and community resources to support patients experiencing insurance denials and appeals, gender marker and name changes, and discrimination in housing, employment, and other sectors.

Nongendered Language

Nongendered language is recommended when referring to anatomy and body processes until the patient identifies the best terms for their provider to use [10, 15, 35]. For example, instead of saying "penis" or "vagina" one can say "genitalia." Instead of saying "testes' 'or "ovaries" use the term "gonads." Additional nongendered language includes people with testes/ovaries, testosterone/estrogen-dominant puberty, people who menstruate, and a pregnant person. Terminology that associates sex or gender with specific anatomy should be avoided unless this is the patient's request, i.e., avoid use of male/female reproductive organs; biologically male/female; and vulva/penis. Share the reason you are asking about a specific body part: "We are going to explore the health of this area so I am going to ask you about it - what term should I use?" Patients' names or terms for sensitive body parts should be elicited in the intake process or during the physical exam. Always follow the patient's lead. Patient-centered language decouples anatomy from the culturally constructed binary gendered experience and honors the patient's self-knowledge as well as the vast diversity of human bodies and gender.

Exploring Provider Bias

Gender impacts all patients differently and as such, providers are tasked with supporting the diversity of patients that seek their professional care. To achieve this, providers and staff members need to inspect their own biases and internal beliefs about gender diversity, including the endociscentric perspective that endocisgender bodies are "normal," and gender expansive bodies are not. This belief is deeply rooted in bias and a pathologization of the diversity of gender experience. The Gender Affirmative Clinical Model clearly states that gender diversity is not a disorder [32, 36]. All bodies, all genders, deserve competent, culturally sensitive care.

Gender Inclusive Clinic Spaces

Gender inclusive clinic spaces can increase patient comfort and satisfaction as well as decrease the experiences of discrimination and stigma experienced by TGNBI patients. These spaces support patients of all genders in accessing the healthcare their bodies need and are discussed at greater length in the next section. The TGNBI community should be instrumental in determining how your space can become more inclusive.

Policies and Procedures

Office policies and procedures should include gender affirming intake processes, all gender facility access, and gender informed customer service/human resources procedures that guide staff in addressing patient and/or staff complaints about discrimination or experiences of misgendering. Each of these are discussed in upcoming sections; examples of policies and procedures can be found in Appendix 1.

Gender Affirming Systems Audit List

Due to staff turnover and the continuous evolution of gender care, a yearly audit of gender affirming systems, including physical office spaces, virtual office space, training practices, and clinic policy and procedures is recommended. The Gender Affirming Clinic Assessment Tool, developed by JM Jaffe, is a resource for clinics to conduct gender affirming systems audits and can be accessed through their website [see Appendix 1 (3) for access instructions].

Creating Inclusive Clinical Spaces

Clinic Entrance

Gender inclusive signs or images posted at the clinic entrance, whether on an external door or a door in a suite of offices, clearly communicate acknowledgment and support of gender diversity. Braille inscription can be added. Some examples of signage are: "All Genders Welcome" or "This is a gender affirming space." To

13 Creating Inclusive, Gender Affirming Clinical Environments

further celebrate inclusion, there are many flags that represent gender diversity—the transgender flag, the agender flag, the nonbinary flag, the genderqueer flag, the intersex flag, and more [37]. These clearly communicate that the clinic welcomes gender diverse patients and may help lessen distress, fear, or hesitation related to seeking services [38]. This is especially important in settings that have traditionally been known as "women's health." The inclusion of both the rainbow flag and the transgender flag honors both sexual and gender diversity.

Waiting Room and Other Clinic Spaces

Signage that communicates gender inclusivity should be displayed in the waiting room along with clinic non-discrimination and inclusion policies. Signs asking patients about their pronouns are recommended in the waiting room, as well as in each room of the clinic. As an example, the "We want to know your pronouns" signs from the Student Health Center at the University of California, Santa Cruz (Fig. 13.3) can be modified for each clinic area. Note that the term "preferred pronouns" is no longer used. Some individuals will have multiple pronouns, such as both he/him and they/them (he/they), or no pronouns and just use their name instead of pronouns.

There should be a range of visual images on the waiting room walls, with diverse images representing different genders, races, ethnicities, sexual orientations, body

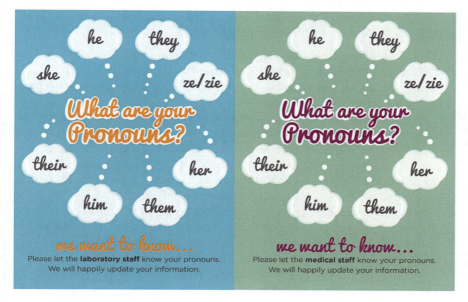

Fig. 13.3 Examples of "we want to know your pronouns" UCSC Health Center (with permission)

sizes, and abilities [[38] verify same as previous citation]. Binary, gender-based color schemes, such as blue and pink walls should be avoided.

The books and magazines that are available for patients to look at in each part of the clinic should be inclusive of the TGNBI community. Some examples of materials to include are: children's books that explore the diversity of gender identities and expressions; pamphlets and brochures on health including binding, tucking, hormone therapy, and gender inclusive sex education; as well as resources for cisgender parents, caregivers, and family members. Appropriate posters and pamphlets should be available in clinic rooms to provide patients and providers with visual reminders of the wide range of transgender and intersex bodies. See Appendices 3 and 4 for a list of pamphlets, educational brochures, children's books, and other written materials and resources.

Restrooms

TGNBI individuals have the right to access the restroom that makes them feel most safe. Exclusionary restroom policies and lack of accommodations have led to traumatization of this community and contribute to heightened vulnerability, fear, and anxiety. This often results in increased stigma and risk of physical violence. Due to lack of safe access to restrooms, TGNBI individuals disproportionately avoid using public restrooms for long periods of time which results in disproportionately high rates of urinary tract and kidney infections, constipation, and other health issues [1, 39, 40]. Clinic environments can create safer and inclusive restroom access for all people by implementing the following policies and practices:

1. Ensure that your clinic includes transgender inclusive policies that allow people of all genders to use the restroom that aligns with their gender experience.
2. Clearly display the gender inclusive restroom policy outside of and inside each restroom.
3. If the facility has only one single-occupancy restroom, consider changing the restroom sign to "Restroom" or "Restroom for Everyone" (Fig. 13.4). Single stall, all gender restrooms increase privacy and decrease stigma and discrimination for transgender and nonbinary individuals [41]. An increasing number of states, including California and Massachusetts, have legislated that *all* single-stall restrooms be designated as gender neutral restrooms [42].
4. If the facility has more than 2 multi-stall restrooms, consider turning one or more of them into a gender neutral restroom. Facilities can either maintain them as multi-stall for all genders to use or convert them to a single-occupancy restroom by installing an "occupied/unoccupied" lock on the external door.
5. If the facility has only "male" and "female" multi-stall restrooms, post signs to make existing restrooms more inclusive and state where an all-gender restroom is located. An example of such signage is: *"Gender diversity is welcomed and respected here. All are welcome to use the restroom that best fits their identity. Single stall restrooms are located at the following locations: _."*

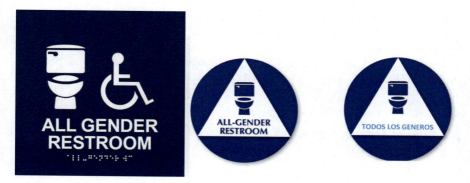

Fig. 13.4 Examples of all gender restroom signs (public domain)

6. If the clinic is in a suite and part of a larger building or set of suites, make sure that restrooms that are in the spaces that are shared by other offices have clear signage of gender inclusive policies, and provide gender inclusive outreach and education to adjacent offices.
7. Provide menstrual products and disposal containers in all restrooms.
8. Include other languages as appropriate, and Braille in all signage.
9. Provide training for staff, emphasizing why taking steps to increase restroom access is essential to creating and maintaining a gender inclusive clinic space. Staff and patients should have opportunities for ongoing dialogue to address any concerns staff and patients may have. For example, some stalls may have doors with large gaps, easily seen through. A solution for this is purchasing privacy covers to cover these gaps.

Telehealth

Providing virtual gender care has become an important priority for medical and mental health/social service entities with the rapid rise in the use of telehealth and telemedicine platforms. The global spread of COVID-19 catapulted most behavioral and physical health providers and organizations to provide services via telehealth.

The basic principles of creating welcoming, gender affirming clinical environments also apply to the virtual world. Awareness of language and pronouns is essential for all staff at every point of contact. When using virtual platforms, ensure that pronouns are part of each staff person's screen name so that pronouns are clearly visible everywhere names are visible, and include accommodations such as options for sign language and captions for the hearing impaired. Staff pronouns also need to be included in the signature stamps of written and email communications.

For virtual visits, including phone calls, it is recommended that all staff verbally introduce themselves with their name and pronouns, and confirm the patient's chosen name and pronouns. With phone calls it is particularly important to not make assumptions based on voice pitch. These practices are recommended for all patients and all clinical visits, not just for TGNBI patients and visits.

Electronic Health Records

Overview

Electronic health record (EHR) systems suffer from the lack of a standardized process for data collection, storage, and retrieval of gender related information for reporting and clinical purposes. An ideal EHR system should be able to capture the full complexity of gender. Although most EHR vendors have been working on gender inclusive modifications, data collection can vary even within the same EHR system at different institutions. This poses a significant barrier to providing quality healthcare to TGNBI patients [43]. Reconciling the differing recommendations for EHR implementation can be complex. Clinics will typically need administrative involvement to advocate for changes in the EHR. Increasingly, health insurers as well as state and federal agencies are requiring clinics to collect more gender specific data to inform program and policy development. EHR systems are undergoing rapid change, but thus far have been unable to match the pace of change in affirming terminology and data requirements in the field of gender affirmed care.

Demographic Data Collection

Current best practice recommendations for collecting a patient's gender demographic data include chosen name, legal name, legal sex; name and sex associated with insurance; sex assigned at birth, and gender identity [43]. EHR systems vary in which gender demographic data fields are used and how they are used. Many systems use terms inappropriately, for example, using the terms sex and gender interchangeably. Some systems require sex designated at birth while others require current legal sex. Either can potentially result in incorrect health screening recommendations, incorrect laboratory interpretations, and/or unsuccessful insurance billing for those whose gender listed in the EHR does not align with the service provided [44].

For example, consider a transgender man who was "assigned female at birth," has not had surgeries, whose legal sex has been changed to "M" (male) and uses he/him pronouns. He is prescribed testosterone and his provider orders testosterone levels. If the EHR uses his assigned sex (F), his lab results will be interpreted incorrectly with (endosex/cis) "female" normed values rather than (endosex/cis) "male" normed

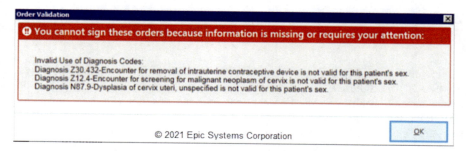

Fig. 13.5 Screenshot of electronic medical record preventing documentation and billing for IUD removal and cervical examination based on male (M) marker [from Epic Systems Corporation]

values, and the results will be flagged as "abnormal" even if they are in fact well within a "normal" range for a person with his hormonal milieu. If the EHR indicates his legal sex as "M" (male) and does not have a mechanism for taking into account his cervix, uterus, or ovaries, his clinician may not recognize his need for cervical cancer screening or inquire about his interest in contraceptive methods appropriate for his anatomy. Further, the EHR would not have a way to document or bill his cervical screening or intrauterine device (IUD) placement or removal (Fig. 13.5).

Additionally, if the patient needs a gender affirming surgical intervention, such as a hysterectomy, being listed as male in the EHR can result in denial by his insurance, as health insurers will often require gender categories for procedures. Ultimately, removing gender and sex categories from billing and coding requirements would simplify and remove barriers to quality care for TGNBI as well as endosex, cisgender individuals.

It is recommended that the patient's chosen name(s) and pronouns be in a prominent, consistent place in the electronic record banner so that every staff person interacting with the patient is cued to use their correct name and pronouns [15, 43]. At registration and intake, patients should have an opportunity to share and update their pronouns and names.

If a person's chosen name(s) and name associated with their insurance are different, these should be captured in distinct fields to support both a successful visit for the patient and the billing process. Note that the name linked with insurance may not be the person's current legal name or chosen name; "legal" name actually has limited clinical and administrative utility.

Name, sex, and gender fields also populate letters and forms generated by the EHR. Review the process by which healthcare maintenance/screening reminders are generated for preventive care such as cervical cancer and mammography screenings. Assure that appropriate persons are identified for screenings which are based on anatomy present and sex hormone milieu. Verify that there is a process for identifying the correct name for outgoing mail. Using nongendered language can simplify all written communication including patient education handouts, consent forms and letters, and reduce the chance of misgendering patients.

SOGI(E): Sexual Orientation, Gender Identity (Gender Expression)

Collecting sexual orientation and gender identity data, known in the United States as "SOGI" or "SOGIE" (including gender expression) is recommended as part of the electronic health record. International journals describe similar content as "GSSO" referring to gender (identity), sex (assigned at birth), and sexual orientation [44]. In the United States, SOGI collection was initially recommended in 2011 by the Institute of Medicine and the Joint Commission. As of 2016, all federally funded health centers are required to collect and report SOGI data annually. A Uniform Data System (UDS) records this data. In 2018, the Centers for Medicare and Medicaid Services required that all electronic health records have the ability to record SOGI as part of Meaningful Use accreditation.

There is consensus on the importance of collecting SOGI data to identify, document, and address LGBTQI (Lesbian, Gay, Bisexual, Transgender, Queer, Questioning and Intersex) health disparities to improve care and support quality research. However, variability in how the data is collected, where data is located in the EHR, and lack of staff training continue to hamper SOGI data collection [44]. SOGI is often embedded in sections of the health record that are not easily accessible or consistently used. Even with the best SOGI collection systems and provider training, clinicians do not always take the time to complete or seek out SOGI data. Some healthcare entities and providers have been reluctant to collect SOGI data for fear of offending patients or of not being able to respond in a gender affirming way. However, research shows that patients support SOGI collection, especially if the reasons for collecting SOGI are shared, and that asking these questions do not alienate patients who are not LGBTQI [13, 43]. With practice and ongoing training, staff become comfortable and reasonably competent with the SOGI process [45].

The current UDS-recommended process for collecting gender data as part of SOGI involves a "two-step" registration process that queries gender identity first, then sex assigned at birth. The question, "What was your sex assigned at birth?" was added to increase accuracy and rates of identifying transgender patients as compared to the previous one-step method, with choices of "male," "female," or "transgender" [46]. There is increasing awareness that the phrase "sex assigned at birth," which implies genetic sex but is based only on appearance of external genitalia, has limited clinical or scientific utility, does not reliably capture relevant clinical information regarding anatomy present or transition history, is not reliably inclusive of intersex patients, and is increasingly stressful to TGNBI patients [47, 48]. An alternative proposal is to refer to the information from gender identity, the organ inventory, and surgical and procedure history to determine the information that one would get by asking sex assigned at birth.

Patients have been critical of the limited choices in terminology in SOGI and want a wider range of sexuality and gender identifiers. Patients also want to be able to indicate more than one sexuality and/or gender [49]. In response, some programs have developed expanded options for both sexual orientation and gender identity, with the ability to "select all that apply" in addition to the open-ended fields that can be filled out (Fig. 13.6). If using expanded SOGI terminology, a process is needed to map the additional terms into the UDS framework for reporting purposes.

13 Creating Inclusive, Gender Affirming Clinical Environments

How would you describe your sexuality? (Check all that apply)

- ☐ Lesbian
- ☐ Gay
- ☐ Bisexual
- ☐ Queer
- ☐ Pansexual
- ☐ Heterosexual (Straight)
- ☐ Not Listed: _____

- ☐ Dyke
- ☐ Faggot
- ☐ Same Gender Loving
- ☐ Asexual (Ace)
- ☐ Aromantic (Aro)
- ☐ Demisexual

- ☐ BDSM/Kink
- ☐ Skoliosexual
- ☐ T4T (trans for trans)
- ☐ Questioning
- ☐ I don't use labels

How would you describe your gender identity? (Check all that apply):

- ☐ Woman
- ☐ Man
- ☐ MTF
- ☐ FTM
- ☐ Trans Feminine
- ☐ Trans Masculine
- ☐ Transguy
- ☐ Feminine-of-Center
- ☐ Masculine-of-Center
- ☐ T-Girl
- ☐ T-Boy
- ☐ Not Listed: _____

- ☐ Trans
- ☐ Transgender
- ☐ Transsexual
- ☐ Femme
- ☐ Butch
- ☐ Stud
- ☐ Aggressive (AG)
- ☐ Boi
- ☐ Androgynous
- ☐ Demigirl
- ☐ Demiboy

- ☐ Tomboy
- ☐ Two-Spirit
- ☐ Hijra
- ☐ Kathoey
- ☐ Muxe
- ☐ Khanith
- ☐ Gender Non-Conforming
- ☐ Genderqueer
- ☐ Gender Variant
- ☐ Gender Fluid

- ☐ Non-Binary
- ☐ Genderfuck
- ☐ Bi-Gender
- ☐ Multi-Gender
- ☐ Pangender
- ☐ Gender Creative
- ☐ Gender Expansive
- ☐ Third Gender
- ☐ Agender/Neutrois
- ☐ Questioning
- ☐ Don't use labels

Fig. 13.6 Example of expanded SOGI from Lyon-Martin Health Services—example of expanded options, multiple choices allowed, without the question "what sex where you assigned at birth?" Link for complete intake form in Appendix 1 (4)

In order to increase patient comfort and disclosure, patients should be provided a confidential setting, such as an online portal, to complete SOGI data. Some patients may wait to share SOGI information until they are meeting with a clinician or until after they feel safe with the clinician [15]. Discussing the confidentiality of gender and sexuality information is an important part of establishing safety. Ideally, there should be a mechanism to ensure that gender information is not shared without explicit consent (unless there are issues of abuse or potential harm to self). Unfortunately, there are not always clear ways to protect some parts of the medical record. Some patients will need confidentiality for employment, family, or other reasons.

There are varying state requirements regarding disclosure for youth. It is important to discuss this with youth who may not yet be "out" to their parents or guardians. If the patient is a minor, be sure to let the youth know that parents may have access to the paperwork that shows name and gender. Familiarity with state requirements and medical record functionality where a given provider practices is crucial for patient safety.

Affirming Patient Encounters

Inclusive Histories, Review of Systems, Body Inventory

Patient intake processes should use a gender inclusive template for all patients, regardless of gender. Using the same template for all patients avoids the issue of staff incorrectly determining which form a patient should fill out based on patient appearance or assumed gender identity.

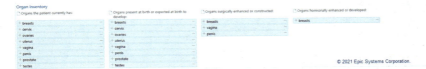

Fig. 13.7 Screenshot of the electronic medical record with organ inventory as part of Transition Summary [from Epic Systems Corporation]. Organs surgically enhanced or constructed leaves out testes

Creating an intake form specifically for TGNBI patients can result in front desk staff making gendered assumptions; these assumptions may result in inaccurate histories and incomplete medical information. For example, if a nonbinary patient who has a male (M) gender marker in the chart is given an intake form designed for endosex cisgender men, this person will not be prompted to share possible menstrual, pregnancy, abortion, menopausal, or surgical history which may be relevant to the patient's body experience. Individuals may or may not have the anatomy assumed to be associated with their gender marker. Using a universal intake form, regardless of gender identity, allows for confidential disclosure and can increase the accuracy in patient reporting, especially among those in the process of coming out or those who do not wish to disclose their gender identity as part of SOGI, or at all.

Intake forms should include a review of systems; medical, surgical, family, gender, and sexual histories; personal language for body parts; and an anatomy or "body" inventory, referred to as an "organ inventory" in the literature (Fig. 13.7). Designating anatomy present, surgical history, and history of hormone use is a recommended best practice and decreases the potential labor, stigma, and distress many patients experiences when they have to disclose information about body parts or characteristics that are not included in the intake process. A body inventory as part of intake further increases accuracy of clinical information [10, 44, 46] and, as discussed above, in conjunction with information from the gender history may ultimately replace the question "sex assigned at birth."

Ideally, the body inventory data populates appropriate clinical guidance and workflows, including healthcare maintenance in the EHR. For example, an intersex transgender man, depending on his anatomy and sexual behaviors and desires, may or may not need cervical cancer or STI screening, abortion care, fertility and pregnancy support or pregnancy prevention, including emergency contraception. There are similar issues and challenges for patients of any gender who may or may not have had gender affirming surgeries or other medical interventions that are not assessed in traditional intake processes.

Beyond SOGI: Sexual Histories

SOGI is not designed to elicit specific details of sexual activity or behavior that are fundamental to supporting patient health. In addition to acknowledging that patients and partners may have multiple and diverse sexual identities, sexual histories need

13 Creating Inclusive, Gender Affirming Clinical Environments

an inclusive framework that transcends labels and includes the body parts and organs present for the patient and their partners or partner, as well as how these body parts, organs, and related fluids interact. This will increase the accuracy of population risk calculations for infection or unintended pregnancy for a patient. As an example, a common assumption by providers is that lesbian sexuality involves two endosex cisgender women, with a lowered risk of STI, and no chance of either becoming pregnant through their exclusive sexual activity. With this narrow definition of what being a lesbian is (recall that a woman may have a vagina or a penis or both or something else), actual infection and unintended pregnancy risks are obfuscated. Suggestions for gender inclusive sexual history scripts can include, *"Sexual health is part of overall health. In order for me to assess your sexual health, I need to know what parts and fluids are involved and what parts and fluids go where* [10, 50].

In summary, make sure that all intake forms are inclusive of all genders, with expanded options for designating multiple gender identities, multiple sexual orientations, and actual sexual behavior. This supports accurate and complete data accrual, increased accuracy in assessment of health risks, and the ability to provide appropriate reproductive and preventive healthcare recommendations. Refer to the Lyon-Martin Health Services intake form as an example; a link to the form is found in Appendix 1 (4).

Physical Exam

In order to provide a patient-centered physical exam, it is important to have an awareness of pacing, relational spacing, and psychological dynamics. Slow down, check-in, integrate shared decision-making for physical exams and procedures, normalize diverse anatomy, and offer specific trauma-informed supportive approaches during sensitive exams or cervical cancer screening. The high rates of sexual assault, medical trauma, dysphoria, testosterone-induced vaginal atrophy, and other causes of physical discomfort with exams highlight the need for increased sensitivity and training on the part of providers and support staff.

Again, awareness of language is paramount, including using nongendered language and removing words with sexual connotation ("let your legs drop to either side" rather than "open up your legs.") Using nongendered descriptors, such as "genitalia" or "external genitalia" instead of "penis" or "vagina" (more examples in the training section) and eliciting patients' personal language for relevant body parts during exams increase patient comfort [35, 51]. Personal language can be elicited during intake as part of the patient history, with the provider before the physical exam, or when discussing recommended preventive care. For example, during cervical cancer screening, use patient-identified or nongendered language such as "genital opening" instead of vagina. The diversity of replacement terms for "vagina" is shown in a word cloud (Fig. 13.8), although some of these are terms that are used with intimate partners, most likely not with medical providers.

Inclusive templates for physical exams that include the full range of organs and anatomy are important for accurate documentation. Gendered exam

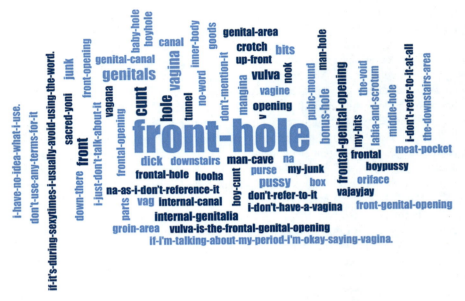

Fig. 13.8 Word Cloud for personal replacement terms provided by TGNBI people for "vagina" within a national online sexual and reproductive health survey (May to September 2019, United States n = 1704). APHA Conference presentation Sachiko Ragosta, October 27, 2020. "From "shark-week" to "mangina": Preferred words reported for sexual and reproductive health anatomy by transgender, non-binary and gender-expansive people"

templates limit accurate documentation. A traditional endocis male exam template does not permit documentation of body parts present for someone who has a vagina, uterus, and ovaries; likewise, a traditional endocis female exam template does not allow documentation of testes or penis. An inclusive, unlabeled anatomical drawing that can be modified dependent on anatomy present, as shown in Fig. 13.9, is a useful adjunct to medical record templates. If you have images of genitalia as part of your practice, offer more than the typical binary penis and vulva. Include images or drawings of nonbinary and intersex genitalia that reflect and normalize diversity such as a vulva with enlarged clitoris/phallus, vaginoplasty, and phalloplasty [35].

13 Creating Inclusive, Gender Affirming Clinical Environments

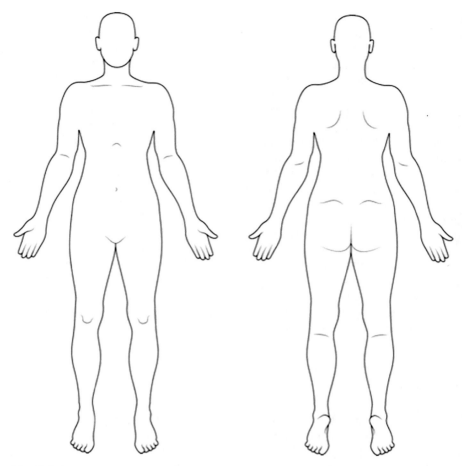

Fig. 13.9 Example of template for nongendered diagram for physical exam (permission granted Katya Tetzlaff)

Billing and Insurance Issues

According to Section 1557 of the Affordable Care Act, "individuals cannot be denied healthcare or health coverage based on their sex, including their gender identity" [52]. This statute means that patients must be treated and addressed in a way consistent with their gender identity, including providing: (1) access to gender-segregated facilities; (2) sex-specific healthcare services that cannot be denied or limited just because the person is a different gender (for example, a provider or insurance company may not deny treatment for ovarian cancer based on an individual's experience as a transgender man or M gender marker); (3) explicit categorical exclusions of coverage for services related to gender transition are facially discriminatory (for example, if the insurance company covers mastectomy to treat breast cancer, then they must also cover it to treat gender dysphoria). State laws vary greatly, but currently 22 states have explicit non-discrimination laws mandating coverage of medically necessary transition-related care for Medicaid plans, and 24 states have non-discrimination legislation for commercial plans [53, 54].

Despite the existence of Section 1557 and state non-discrimination laws, coverage for gender care, such as hormones, surgeries, hair removal, and voice therapy, continues to vary greatly depending on state laws, insurance company, insurance plan, and the individual handling the request for coverage. In addition to specifically gender affirming care, TGNBI patients continue to be excluded from or denied appropriate healthcare because insurance companies often have automatic denials when the patient's anatomy does not correlate to their gender marker (for example, pap smears, pelvic ultrasounds, birth control or mammograms for someone with a male gender marker or a prostate exam for someone with a female gender marker). Thus, it is important for clinicians and support staff to learn how to navigate the appeals process to ensure gender diverse patients are able to access the medically necessary care they need [55]. One tip for avoiding denials is to include Condition Code 45 to procedure and visit codes in which the gender marker and procedure or diagnosis is likely to be perceived by the plan as an error. Condition code 45 alerts the plan that the gender/procedure or gender/diagnosis "conflict" is not an error, allowing the claim to be processed without interruption. For more information on insurance, billing, and navigating insurance denials, see specific resources in Appendix 5.

Marketing

All advertising materials need to be reviewed and revised for gender inclusivity. If photographs are used, source TGNBI sites that provide stock photos (The Gender Spectrum Collection by Broadly, as an example) or pay TGNBI individuals to be depicted in photos. Gendered language and imagery should be removed from all marketing and descriptive materials [10]. For example, the words "woman" or "man" can be replaced with "person" or "persons." Clinic websites should include descriptions of gender affirming medical services and include pronouns in all staff bios as well as the specific role each staff member has in supporting TGNBI patients. Including specific experience in providing gender care is recommended. Marketing and outreach materials should be reviewed by the Community Advisory Board before publishing.

Moving Forward

Providing high quality, gender affirming care is both a challenge and a profound honor. Key recommendations, touching on facilities, patient-facing materials, and clinical encounters are highlighted in Table 13.1 ["Recommendations for Building

Table 13.1 Recommendations for building gender inclusive clinical settings, modified with permission from Moseson, et al. The Imperative for Transgender and Nonbinary Inclusion, Obstetrics and Gynecology, 2020

Context	Marginalizing practices	Inclusive practices
Clinical facilities	"Women" in titles, signage, e.g., "Women's Health Clinic."	Describe the nature of care provided, e.g., "Reproductive Health Clinic."
	Gendered bathrooms (men's room and women's room)	Single stall bathrooms should be all gender: "Restroom" or "All Gender Restroom." If only multi stall bathrooms available, at least one should be marked "All Gender Restroom."
	"Women's" vs "men's" waiting area	Offer all gender waiting areas or offer private waiting areas.
	Inflexibility in appointment times without regard to patient preferences and needs.	Flexibility in offering patient appointments at the very beginning or end of the shift if a patient has concerns about their safety and/or comfort in the waiting area.
	"Breastfeeding room" or "Mother's room"	"Nursing parents' room" or "Infant feeding room"
	Marketing sexual and reproductive health services to people assigned female at birth only.	Offer sexual and reproductive health services for everyone with marketing to all genders—e.g., affirming STI testing and care, general health screening, and fertility preservation. Use nongendered language in describing services; replace "women" with "persons" or "people" in descriptive brochures.
Paperwork, patient education	Pictures of cisgender women (or cisgender heterosexual couples) used to illustrate contraception, abortion, or pregnancy.	Include pictures of pregnant people of all genders (cisgender women, transgender, and nonbinary people); include people who are in same gender partnerships.
	Using pink, flowers, and butterflies to advertise health services.	Avoid unnecessarily gendering care in design schemes and avoid traditional markers of femininity.

(continued)

Table 13.1 (continued)

Context	Marginalizing practices	Inclusive practices
Clinical encounters	Using gender or sex-specific intake forms.	Use the same, all gender, intake form for all patients, without questions designated as for "women only" or "men only." Use an all gender intake form that asks people to indicate the organs they have and solicits words that each patient uses to talk about their body parts, to guide patient and provider interactions. See Lyon-Martin Health Services intake form with link in Appendix. All intake forms should receive input from a diverse cross-section of patient representatives or community board.
	Asking only for legal name and sex	At registration, ask every patient, regardless of assumed gender identity, for their affirmed name and pronouns. Note this information clearly in the patient file or EHR and assure that all staff use it throughout the clinical encounter. For gender identity, offer multiple options: Man, woman, nonbinary, genderqueer, transgender, or another gender not specified, and include a write-in option. Allow patients to indicate the name and sex that is registered with their insurance, legal name and sex, and anatomy/organs that they currently have. Verify this information at subsequent visits, as name, gender identity, pronouns, and legal/administrative sex may change. Educate and train staff so that they understand the importance of and are comfortable with asking this information.
	Rely on patients to offer pronouns	Create a culture in which clinic staff introduce themselves with their pronouns ("Hi, I'm Dr. J and my pronouns are she and her. How are you today?") and include pronouns on staff identification badges. If not assessed on forms or prior to encounter, ask patient's name and pronouns: "What name do you want me to use? What are your pronouns?"
	Not using collected information on pronouns/identity, or recording this information in a place that is difficult to reference	Store patient pronouns and identity information in a place that is visible and readily accessible to all staff who need to identify or communicate with the patient, throughout each encounter and from encounter-to-encounter. Ideally, wherever the patient's name is displayed, the identified pronouns are also visible.
	Assume which body parts or organs a person might have based on gender identity or sex assigned at birth	Ask or assess all patients (with intake forms etc.) the body parts or organs they have in systematic way, regardless of gender identity and record this in a way that is accessible to other clinicians from encounter to encounter.

Assume use of clinical terms for body parts	Ask all patients which terms they prefer to use to describe their own body parts, and whether there are any terms they are not comfortable using, regardless of gender identity. Demonstrate awareness of when and where language may not be ideal—e.g., "I'm going to use anatomical terms because that's the clearest way that I can describe this;" or "This pamphlet refers to all pregnant people as women, but it has some really helpful information about X."
Assume particular pregnancy or fertility desires of transgender or gender nonbinary patients	Introduce the topic of pregnancy and family building neutrally, without assuming anything about pregnancy or fertility preservation desires, and discuss all related options including contraception, pregnancy, parenting, abortion, adoption, co-housing, co-parenting, and more.
Asking only about "opposite" (or assumed opposite) gender when taking sexual histories	In taking sexual history for all genders, ask patients to specify the gender identities and body parts of partners. Do not make assumptions of body parts based on gender identity, names, or pronouns. and allow patients to specify the gender(s) and body parts of partners. Ask additional questions as necessary to clarify partners' anatomy and specific sexual behaviors.
Require patients to remove clothes for much of the appointment	Conduct as much of the appointment as possible with patient clothes on and allow patients the opportunity to defer invasive physical exams to another appointment (unless patient requests exam or absolutely necessary).
Training only direct clinical providers in gender affirming practices	Work with ancillary providers (e.g., pharmacists and radiographers) as well as other facility staff with patient contact (receptionists, phone operators, billing and insurance staff, etc.) to make sure that every step of the care pathway is welcoming.
Use of gendered terms for routine care (i.e., "well woman's exam")	Describe exams and procedures in nongendered ways, such as "preventative care visit" or "pelvic exam" or "contraceptive services," or "cervical cancer screening".

Gender inclusive Clinical Settings"]. While specific recommendations will change, the core values of listening with humility, respect, and an openness to change can guide clinic systems and providers in continuing to create environments where patients feel safe and receive quality reproductive healthcare. The creation and maintenance of an inclusive, gender affirming clinical environment is a dynamic process that demands openness and ongoing assessment as this field continues to change rapidly.

Appendix 1: Resources for Developing Gender Affirming Clinical Environments

1. Fenway Institute—The National LGBT Health Education Center-many relevant offerings (https://www.lgbtqiahealtheducation.org/resources/in/organizational-change/type/publication/).
   (a) "Affirmative Services for Transgender and Gender Diverse People - Best Practices for Frontline Healthcare Staff"
   (b) "The Nuts and Bolts of SOGI Implementation: A Troubleshooting Toolkit"
   (c) "Recruiting, Training, and Retaining LGBTQ-Proficient Clinical Providers: A Workforce Development Toolkit"
   (d) "Creating a Transgender Health Program at Your Health Center"
   (e) "Fact Sheet: Transgender Health and Medical Legal Partnerships"
   (f) "LGBT Health Readiness Assessments in Health Centers: Key Findings"
   (g) "Focus on Forms and Policy: Creating an Inclusive Environment for LGBT Patients"
2. The Teaching Transgender Toolkit, E. Greene & L. Maurer (http://www.teachingtransgender.org).
3. The Gender affirming Clinical Assessment Tool (http://transhealthconsulting.com) *Password protected link to the assessment tool:* TGIHealthcareTA (no fee with this password).
4. Lyon Martin Health Services intake form: /https://transline.zendesk.com/hc/en-us/articles/229380508-Lyon-Martin-s-Intake-Forms
5. American Medical Association: Creating an LGBTQ-friendly Practice; (https://www.ama-assn.org/delivering-care/population-care/creating-lgbtq-friendly-practice).
6. Human Rights Campaign: Transgender Inclusion in the Workplace: A toolkit for Employers. 2016. https://assets2.hrc.org/files/assets/resources/Transgender_Inclusion_in_the_Workplace_A_Toolkit_for_Employers_Version_10_14_2016.pdf
7. Creating Equal Access to Quality Health Care for Transgender Patients: Transgender affirming Hospital Policies [Internet]. New York City, NY: Lambda Legal; 2016 May. Available from: https://www.lambdalegal.org/sites/default/files/publications/downloads/hospital-policies-2016_5-26-16.pdf
8. Kelly M. Providing Transgender and Non-binary Care at Planned Parenthood: A Best Practice Guide and Start-Up Action Kit. 2018.

13 Creating Inclusive, Gender Affirming Clinical Environments

https://maureenkellyconsulting.com/resources-%26-writing

Appendix 2: Training and Other Resources for Providers

1. Fenway Institute—The National LGBT Health Education Center- many CME trainings (https://www.lgbtqiahealtheducation.org/).
2. UCSF Transgender Care and Treatment Guidelines (https://transcare.ucsf.edu/guidelines).
3. Project HEALTH: TransLine (http://project-health.org/transline/).
4. The Teaching Transgender Toolkit, E. Greene & L. Maurer (http://www.teachingtransgender.org).
5. Gender Spectrum: "Establishing Trust with Youth Seeking Gender Affirmative Medical Care" (https://static1.squarespace.com/static/5ac6a3e825bf0250fa23d6cb/t/5b329131575d1ff01744b94d/1530040625617/Establishing+Trust+with+Youth+Seeking+Gender+Affirmative+Medical+Care.pdf).
6. Gender Education Network (https://gendereducationnetwork.com).
7. WPATH GEI: Global Education Initiative (https://www.wpath.org/gei).
8. Chang SC, Singh AA, dickey lore m. A clinician's guide to gender-affirming care: Working with Transgender & gender-nonconforming clients. Oakland, CA: Context Press, an imprint of New Harbinger Publications, Inc.; 2018. *need Vancouver citation format*
9. Shlasko D, Hofius K. Trans allyship workbook: Building skills to support trans people in our lives. Madison, WI: Think Again Training; 2017. *need Vancouver citation format.*
10. Keo-Meier C, Ehrensaft D. The Gender Affirmative Model: An Interdisciplinary Approach to Supporting Transgender and Gender Expansive Children. Columbia, MD: American Psychological Association; 2018. *need Vancouver citation format.*
11. Fielding L. Trans sex: Clinical approaches to trans sexualities and erotic embodiments. Routledge; 2021. (Chapter 6: Bringing Theory into Practice. "Anatomy Talk" by Heather Edwards, PT CSC).
12. Supporting Trans Autistic Youth & Adults: A Guide for Professionals and Families by Finn Gratton *need Vancouver citation format.*
13. WPATH: Standards of Care for the Health of Transsexual, Transgender and Gender Non-Conforming People v 7 (https://www.wpath.org/publications/soc).

Appendix 3: Books for Patients in the Waiting and Clinic Rooms

1. What Makes a Baby by Corey Silverberg (youth book).
2. The Gender Wheel by Maya Christina (youth book).
3. The Boy and the Bindi by Vivek Shraya (youth book).

204 J. Hastings et al.

4. When Aidan Became a Big Brother by Kyle Lukoff and Kaylani Juanita (youth book).
5. Stacey's Not a Girl by Colt Keo-Meier.
6. The Gender Quest Workbook by Rylan Testa, Deborah Coolhart, Jayme Peta (young adult).
7. The Gender Creative Child by Diane Ehrensaft.
8. Beyond the Binary by Alok Vaid-Menon.
9. Families in Transition by Arlen Lev and Andrew Gottlieb.
10. The Transgender Child, A Handbook for Families and Professionals, by Stephanie Brill and Rachel Pepper.
11. Trans Bodies, Trans Selves edited by Laura Erickson-Schroth.
12. Reflective Workbook for Partners of Trans People by DM Maynard.

Appendix 4: Pamphlets and Patient Education Handouts for the Waiting and Clinic Rooms

1. The Gender Quest Workbook by Rylan Testa, Deborah Coolhart, Jayme Peta.
2. Somos Familia: https://www.somosfamiliabay.org
3. Trans Youth Family Allies: http://www.imatyfa.org
4. Gender Spectrum: www.genderspectrum.org
   (a) Support Plan & Gender Communication Plan https://genderspectrum.org/articles/using-the-gsp
   (b) Lounge/Support Groups https://lounge.genderspectrum.org/
5. NCTE Identity Documents Center (https://transequality.org/documents).
6. Supportive Families, Healthy Children - Family Acceptance Project (https://familyproject.sfsu.edu).
7. Transgender violence survivors: A Self Help Guide to Healing and Understanding - FORGE: https://www.acesdv.org/wp-content/uploads/2014/06/Trans-Sexual-Violence-Survivors-Self-Help-Guide.pdf
8. Partners Guide: https://www.pvaz.net/DocumentCenter/View/8967/Transgender-Sexual-Violence-Survivors-Partners-Guide
9. Fenway's self-injection guide (https://fenwayhealth.org/wp-content/uploads/2015/07/COM-1880-trans-health_injection-guide_small_v2.pdf).
10. Callen-Lorde's brochures on tucking, binding, voice training.
    (a) http://callen-lorde.org/graphics/2018/09/HOTT-Safer-Tucking_Final.pdf
    (b) http://callen-lorde.org/graphics/2018/09/Safer-Binding_2018_FINAL.pdf
    (c) http://callen-lorde.org/graphics/2018/09/HOTT-Voice-Brochure_Final.pdf
11. TransLine's brochure on silicone pumping: https://transline.zendesk.com/hc/en-us/articles/229372988-TransLine-s-Silicone-Pumping-Safety-Handout
12. PREP pamphlets:
    (a) For transgender and nonbinary people (UK): https://i-base.info/guides/wp-content/uploads/2019/11/UK-guide-to-PrEP-Nov-2019-FINAL.pdf
    (b) For transwomen https://www.poz.com/pdfs/prep_trans_project_inform.pdf

13 Creating Inclusive, Gender Affirming Clinical Environments

13. Safer Sex for Trans Bodies (Whitman Walker & HRC) https://www.hrc.org/resources/safer-sex-for-trans-bodies
14. Nonbinary resources: https://genderqueer.me/resources/

Appendix 5: Billing and Insurance Resources

1. "Supporting Your Patient in Appealing an Insurance Denial" poster by Gill Blasdel and JM Jaffe. (https://static1.squarespace.com/static/599f136a6b8f5b8e60707a05/t/5d89498e4222875f9387cd78/1569278363216/AppealLettersPoster.pdf)
2. Trans Line Insurance Guide (https://transhealthproject.org).
3. Know Your Rights: Health Care (https://transequality.org/health-coverage-guide).

References

1. James SE, Herman JL, Rankin S, Keisling M, Mottet L, Anafi M. The report of the 2015 U. S. Transgender survey. Washington, DC: National Center for Transgender Equality; 2016.
2. Stroumsa D, Kirkland AR. Health coverage and care for transgender people—threats and opportunities. N Engl J Med. 2020;383(25):2397–9.
3. White Hughto JM, Reisner SL, Pachankis JE. Transgender stigma and health: a critical review of stigma determinants, mechanisms, and interventions. Soc Sci Med. 2015;147:222–31.
4. Kcomt L, Gorey KM, Barrett BJ, McCabe SE. Healthcare avoidance due to anticipated discrimination among transgender people: a call to create trans-affirmative environments. SSM Popul Health. 2020;11:100608.
5. Testa RJ, Rider GN, Haug NA, Balsam KF. Gender confirming medical interventions and eating disorder symptoms among transgender individuals. Health Psychol. 2017;36(10):927–36.
6. Méndez JE. Report of the Special Rapporteur on torture and other cruel, inhuman or degrading treatment or punishment. 2013 Feb.
7. The Associated Press. Japan's Supreme Court upholds transgender sterilization requirement [Internet]. NBC News. 2019 [cited 2020 Dec 23]. https://www.nbcnews.com/feature/nbc-out/japan-s-supreme-court-upholds-transgender-sterilization-requirement-n962721
8. Lowik AJ. Reproducing eugenics, reproducing while trans: the state sterilization of trans people. J GLBT Fam Stud. 2018;14(5):425–45.
9. OHCHR, UN Women, UNAIDS, UNDP, UNFPA, UNICEF, WHO. Eliminating forced, coercive and otherwise involuntary sterilization [Internet]. Who.int. 2014 [accessed 2021 Jan 2]. https://apps.who.int/iris/bitstream/handle/10665/112848/9789241507325_eng.pdf:jsessionid=A463B2BF938393E9BA79466DD4BFAE91?sequence=1
10. Moseson H, Zazanis N, Goldberg E, Fix L, Durden M, Stoeffler A, et al. The imperative for transgender and gender nonbinary inclusion: beyond Women's health: beyond women's health. Obstet Gynecol. 2020;135(5):1059–68.
11. Obedin-Maliver J. Time for OBGYNs to care for people of all genders. J Womens Health (Larchmt). 2015;24(2):109–11.
12. Kaplan RL, El Khoury C, Lize N. Discussions about the health of women should include transgender women. Lancet Public Health. 2018;3(6):e269.

13. Grasso C, McDowell MJ, Goldhammer H, Keuroghlian AS. Planning and implementing sexual orientation and gender identity data collection in electronic health records. J Am Med Inform Assoc. 2019;26(1):66–70.
14. Creating a Transgender Health Program at Your Health Center: From Planning to Implementation [Internet]. National LGBTQIA+ Health Education Center; 2018 Sep. *Accessed 2021 Jan 2.*
15. Bizub B, Allen B. A review of clinical guidelines for creating a gender-affirming primary care practice. WMJ. 2020;119(1):8–15.
16. Ross KA, Castle BG. A culture-centered approach to improving healthy trans-patient–practitioner communication: recommendations for practitioners communicating with Trans individuals. Health Commun. 2017;32(6):730–40.
17. Creating equal access to quality health care for transgender patients: transgender-affirming hospital policies [Internet]. New York City, NY: Lambda Legal; 2016 May.
18. Hagen DB, Galupo MP. Trans* individuals' experiences of gendered language with health care providers: recommendations for practitioners. Int J Transgend. 2014;15(1):16–34.
19. Glick JL, Theall K, Andrinopoulos K, Kendall C. For data's sake: dilemmas in the measurement of gender minorities. Cult Health Sex 1080. 2018;20(12):1362–77. 1437220
20. Brooks H, Llewellyn CD, Nadarzynski T, Pelloso FC, De Souza GF, Pollard A, et al. Sexual orientation disclosure in health care: a systematic review. Br J Gen Pract. 2018;68(668):e187–96.
21. Dolan IJ, Strauss P, Winter S, Lin A. Misgendering and experiences of stigma in health care settings for transgender people. Med J Aust. 2020;212(4):150–1.e1
22. McLemore KA. Experiences with misgendering: identity misclassification of transgender spectrum individuals. Self Identity. 2015;14(1):51–74.
23. Russell ST, Pollitt AM, Li G, Grossman AH. Chosen name use is linked to reduced depressive symptoms, suicidal ideation, and suicidal behavior among transgender youth. J Adolesc Health. 2018;63(4):503–5.
24. The Human Rights Campaign Foundation. Transgender inclusion in the workplace: a toolkit for employers. 2016. Accessed 2020 Dec 29.
25. Transgender Law Center. Model transgender employment policy: negotiating for inclusive workplaces. Accessed 2021 Jan 9.
26. Meyer W III, Bockting WO, Cohen-Kettenis P, Coleman E, Diceglie D, Devor H, et al. The Harry Benjamin International Gender Dysphoria Association's Standards of Care for Gender Identity Disorders, sixth version. J Psychol Human Sex. 2001;13(1):1–30.
27. Rider GN, McMorris BJ, Gower AL, Coleman E, Brown C, Eisenberg ME. Perspectives from nurses and physicians on training needs and comfort working with transgender and gender-diverse youth. J Pediatr Health Care. 2019;33(4):379–85.
28. Thomas DD, Safer JD. A simple intervention raised resident-physician willingness to assist transgender patients seeking hormone therapy. Endocr Pract. 2015;21(10):1134–42.
29. Eisenberg ME, McMorris BJ, Rider GN, Gower AL, Coleman E. "It's kind of hard to go to the doctor's office if you're hated there." a call for gender-affirming care from transgender and gender diverse adolescents in the United States. Health Soc Care Community. 2020;28(3):1082–9.
30. Hanssmann C, Morrison D, Russian E. Talking, gawking, or getting it done: provider trainings to increase cultural and clinical competence for transgender and gender-nonconforming patients and clients. Sex Res Social Policy. 2008;5(1):5–23.
31. Prismic. Gender Spectrum [Internet]. Genderspectrum.org. 2019 [cited 2020 Dec 9]. https://www.genderspectrum.org/articles/understanding-gender
32. Keo-Meier C, Ehrensaft D. The gender affirmative model: an interdisciplinary approach to supporting transgender and gender expansive children. American Psychological Association; 2018.
33. UCSF Transgender Care, Department of Family and Community Medicine, University of California San Francisco. Guidelines for the primary and gender-affirming care of transgender and gender nonbinary people. 2nd ed. Deutsch MB, editor. 2016 Jun.
34. Coleman E, Bockting W, Botzer M, Cohen-Kettenis P, DeCuypere G, Feldman J, et al. Standards of care for the health of transsexual, transgender, and gender-nonconforming people, version 7. Int J Transgend. 2012;13(4):165–232. Version 8 in development

35. Fielding L. Trans sex: clinical approaches to trans sexualities and erotic embodiments. Routledge; 2021. ("Anatomy Talk." Heather Edwards, PT, CSC.)
36. Hidalgo MA, Ehrensaft D, Tishelman AC, Clark LF, Garofalo R, Rosenthal SM, Spack NP, Olson J. The gender affirmative model: what we know and what we aim to learn. Hum Dev. 2013;56:5.
37. Converse A. Gender pride flags and what they mean - Deconforming [Internet]. Deconforming. com. 2019 [cited 2021 Jan 4]. https://deconforming.com/gender-pride-flags/
38. Wilkerson JM, Rybicki S, Barber CA, Smolenski DJ. Creating a culturally competent clinical environment for LGBT patients. J Gay Lesbian Soc Serv. 2011;23(3):376–94.
39. Hardacker CT, Baccellieri A, Mueller ER, Brubaker L, Hutchins G, Zhang JLY, et al. Bladder health experiences, perceptions and knowledge of sexual and gender minorities. Int J Environ Res Public Health. 2019;16(17):3170.
40. Schuster MA, Reisner SL, Onorato SE. Beyond bathrooms—meeting the health needs of transgender people. N Engl J Med 2016;375(2):101–103.
41. Weinhardt LS, Stevens P, Xie H, Wesp LM, John SA, Apchemengich I, et al. Transgender and gender nonconforming youths' public facilities use and psychological well-being: a mixed-method study. Transgend Health. 2017;2(1):140–50.
42. Assembly Bill No. 1732 Single-user Restrooms [Internet]. Sep 29, 2016. from: https://leginfo.legislature.ca.gov/faces/billNavClient.xhtml?bill_id=201520160AB1732
43. Deutsch MB, Buchholz D. Electronic health records and transgender patients—practical recommendations for the collection of gender identity data. J Gen Intern Med. 2015;30(6):843–7.
44. Lau F, Antonio M, Davison K, Queen R, Devor A. A rapid review of gender, sex, and sexual orientation documentation in electronic health records. J Am Med Inform Assoc. 2020;27(11):1774–83.
45. The Fenway Institute and NORC. The Nuts and Bolts of SOGI Data Implementation: a troubleshooting toolkit. 2019.
46. Deutsch MB, Green J, Keatley J, Mayer G, Hastings J, Hall AM, et al. Electronic medical records and the transgender patient: recommendations from the World Professional Association for Transgender Health EMR Working Group. J Am Med Inform Assoc. 2013;20(4):700–3.
47. Dunne MJ, Raynor LA, Cottrell EK, Pinnock WJA. Interviews with patients and providers on transgender and gender nonconforming health data collection in the electronic health record. Transgend Health. 2017;2(1):1–7.
48. Shteyler VM, Clarke JA, Adashi EY. Failed assignments—rethinking sex designations on birth certificates. N Engl J Med. 2020;383(25):2399–401.
49. Moseson H, Lunn MR, Katz A, Fix L, Durden M, Stoeffler A, et al. Development of an affirming and customizable electronic survey of sexual and reproductive health experiences for transgender and gender nonbinary people. PLoS One. 2020;15(5):e0232154.
50. Krempasky C, Harris M, Abern L, Grimstad F. Contraception across the transmasculine spectrum. Am J Obstet Gynecol. 2020;222(2):134–43.
51. Ragosta S. From "shark-week" to "mangina": Preferred words reported for sexual and reproductive health anatomy by transgender, non-binary, and gender-expansive people. 2020 Oct 27.
52. Section 1557 of the patient protection and affordable care act: nondiscrimination in health programs and activities proposed rule. 2010.
53. Proctor K, Haffer SC, Ewald E, Hodge C, James CV. Identifying the transgender population in the Medicare program. Transgend Health. 2016;1(1):250–65.
54. Equality Maps: Healthcare Laws and Policies [Internet]. Movement Advancement Project. [cited 2020 Dec 30]. https://www.lgbtmap.org/equality-maps/healthcare_laws_and_policies
55. Blasdel G, Jaffe JM. Supporting your patient in appealing an insurance denial. Poster Session presented at the United States Professional Association of Transgender Health, Washington, DC. 2019 Sep. https://www.healthytrans.com/appeal-letters

Index

A
American Academy of Pediatrics (AAP), 170
Animal models, 41, 42
Anti-Müllerian hormone (AMH), 34, 51
Antral follicle count (AFC), 51
Assisted reproductive technology (ART), 34, 38, 163

B
Bone mineral density (BMD), 14, 16

C
Clinic entrance, 186
Controlled ovarian stimulation (COS), 51, 53

D
Demographics, 1

E
Electronic health record, 179, 190
    demographic data collection, 190, 191
    sexual orientation and gender identity, 191, 192
Estrogen, 14
Exploring provider bias, 185

F
Fallopian tube, 37
Female sexual function index (FSFI), 130
Feminizing, 11

Fertility preservation (FP), 49, 98, 144, 154
    post pubertal transmasculine, 51–53
    pre pubertal transmasculine, 54, 55
Fertilization, 146

G
Gamete cryopreservation, 146
Gender affirming, 179, 180
Gender affirming hormones (GAHs), 97, 143
Gender-affirming treatment (GAT), 49
    estrogen, 16, 19
    feminizing therapies, 19–23
    hormone therapy, 9
    masculinizing hormone therapy, 10
    medications, 10, 12
    perioperative medication management, 19
    physical changes, 13
    risks, 14, 16
    surgical procedures, 17, 18
    surveillance, 14
    testosterone, 13
    TGNB youth management, 24, 25
Gender diverse youth, 97
Gender expansive, 1, 178, 185
Gender identity, 178, 180, 182, 184, 190, 192
Gender inclusive clinic spaces, 186
Gender non-binary, 179
Genderqueer, 1
Gonadectomy, 143
Gonadotropin-releasing hormone (GnRH), 42
Gonadotropin releasing hormone agonist (GnRHa), 97
Gynecology, 109

© The Editor(s) (if applicable) and The Author(s), under exclusive license to
Springer Nature Switzerland AG 2023
M. B. Moravek, G. de Haan (eds.), *Reproduction in Transgender and Nonbinary Individuals*, https://doi.org/10.1007/978-3-031-14933-7

Index

H
Hiring, 182
Hormone therapy, 9, 134, 135
Human papillomavirus (HPV), 115
Hysterectomy, 110, 112, 113

I
Implantation, 146
Intersex, 183
Intracytoplasmic sperm injection (ICSI), 65
Intrauterine insemination, 67
In vitro fertilization (IVF), 67, 68
In vitro maturation (IVM), 41, 55

L
Legislation, 154
  donor insemination statutes, 155, 156
  establishing parentage, 155
  fertility preservation, 154
  marital presumption, 155

M
Marketing, 198
Masculinizing, 12
Masculinizing hormone therapy, 10
Mastectomy, 143
Metoidioplasty, 18, 113
Microsurgical epididymal sperm extraction
  (MESA), 65

N
Neural tube defects (NTDs), 84
Non-gendered language, 185

O
Obstetrics, 76
Oocyte cryopreservation, 51, 53
Ovarian tissue cryopreservation (OTC), 54

P
Percutaneous epididymal sperm aspiration
  (PESA), 65
Phalloplasty, 18, 143
Polycystic ovary syndrome (PCOS),
  34–36, 50
Postpartum depression (PPD), 91
Preconception, 79

R
Reproductive health, 2, 178, 179, 196
Retroejaculation, 65

S
Sexual desire, 130, 131
Sexual function, 130
Sexual health, 3, 5, 129, 130
Sexually transmitted Infection (STI), 115, 131
Staff considerations, 183, 185

T
Telehealth, 189
Testicular sperm aspiration (TESA), 65
Testicular sperm extraction (TESE), 65
Testosterone, 10, 12, 80
  animal models, 41–43
  assisted reproductive technology, 39–41
  fallopian tubes, 37
  ovaries, 34–36
  pregnancies, 37, 38
  uterus, 36, 37
Transfeminine individuals
  hormone therapy, 133–135
  pre-treatment, 131–133
  satisfaction, 138
  sexual function, 129–131
  surgery, 136, 137
Transfeminine people, 60
  biologic impacts, 61, 62
  cryopreserve sperm, 64
  family building options, 68, 70
  genetically related families, 60
  intrauterine insemination, 67
  partner considerations, 64
  psychological considerations, 63
  sperm collection methods, 64, 65
Transgender and non-binary (TGNB), 1, 3, 4,
  9, 33, 59, 75, 103, 141
  abortion methods, 79
  ACA and health care insurance, 159–161
  barriers to medical care, 142, 143
  birth certificates, 158
  competent reproductive care, 143, 144
  contraception, 91
  cost of fertility treatments, 167, 168
  current medical system, 147–149
  decision-making despite uncertainty,
    168, 169
  delivery, 88, 89
  demographics, 1

Index

ethical and legal considerations, 102, 103
fertility preservation, 169–172
health disparities, 3
identity and mental health, 85, 86
inconsistent legal identification, 157
infertility, 164, 165
language, 78
marginalization, 166
medical considerations, 98–100
minority stress, 77
parenthood desires, 144–147
pelvic exams, 86
postpartum, 90
postpartum depression, 91
preconception, 80
preconception screening, 81–85
pregnancy outcomes, 87
prior negative healthcare experiences, 76, 77
psychosocial considerations, 100, 101
reproductive health, 2, 5
sexual health, 3
testosterone, 80, 81
transphobia, 142
trauma-informed care, 78
Transgender, non-binary, and intersex (TGNBI), 177
Transmasculine, 33, 36, 49, 50

Transmasculine patients
chest care, 114
contraception counseling, 116, 117
genital bleeding, 117–120
gynecologic history, 110
human papilloma virus, 115
hysterectomies, 113
metoidioplasty, 113
pelvic pain, 120–122
phalloplasty, 114
sexually transmitted infection, 115
testosterone, 111, 112
vulvovaginal atrophy, 120
Trans men, 52
Transphobia, 142

U
US transgender survey (USTS), 76
Uterine bleeding, 109, 118

V
Vagina, 109
Vaginoplasty, 143
Venous thromboembolism (VTE), 20, 117

W
Waiting room, 187

Printed in the United States
by Baker & Taylor Publisher Services